ENG/VNG

Core Clinical Concepts in Audiology

Series Editor
Brad Stach, PhD

Basic Audiometry
Editors
James W. Hall III & Virginia Ramachandran

Pure-Tone Audiometry and Masking by Maureen Valente, PhD
Basic Audiometry Learning Manual by Mark DeRuiter, PhD, and Virginia Ramachandran, AuD
Speech Audiometry by Gary D. Lawson, PhD, and Mary E. Peterson, PhD

Electrodiagnostic Audiology
Editors
James W. Hall III & Virginia Ramachandran

Objective Assessment of Hearing by James W. Hall III, PhD, and De Wet Swanepoel, PhD
Otoacoustic Emissions: Principles, Procedures, and Protocols by Sumitrajit Dhar
and James W. Hall III

Cochlear Implants
Editors
Terry Zwolan & Jace Wolfe

Programming Cochlear Implants by Jace Wolfe, PhD, and Erin C. Schafer, PhD
Objective Measures in Cochlear Implants by Michelle L. Hughes, PhD, CCC-A

Vestibular Assessment
Editors
Ken Bouchard & Virginia Ramachandran

Vestibular Learning Manual by Bre L. Myers, AuD
ENG/VNG by Devin L. McCaslin, PhD

ENG/VNG

Devin L. McCaslin
Vanderbilt Bill Wilkerson Center
Division of Vestibular Sciences
Balance Disorders Clinic, Nashville, Tennessee

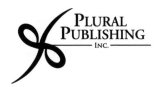

PLURAL
PUBLISHING
INC.

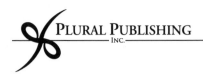

5521 Ruffin Road
San Diego, CA 92123

e-mail: info@pluralpublishing.com
Web site: http://www.pluralpublishing.com

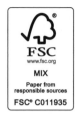

Typeset in 11/13 Palatino by Flanagan's Publishing Services, Inc.
Printed in the United States of America by McNaughton & Gunn
19 18 17 16   4 5 6 7

Library of Congress Cataloging-in-Publication Data

McCaslin, Devin L. (Devin Lochlan)
  Electronystagmography/videonystagmography/Devin L. McCaslin.
     p. ; cm.
  Includes bibliographical references and index.
  ISBN 978-1-59756-412-0 (alk. paper)—ISBN 1-59756-412-5 (alk. paper)
  I. Title.
  [DNLM: 1. Electronystagmography. 2. Eye Movements—physiology. 3. Ocular Motility Disorders—pathology. 4. Oculomotor Muscles—physiology. 5. Vestibular Diseases—diagnosis. 6. Vestibule, Labyrinth—physiopathology. WW 410]

  617.7'62—dc23
                                   2012031492

Contents

Preface

In 1976 a textbook was published that described the quantitative assessment of the vestibular system. This book, *Manual of Electronystagmography*, was written by Hugh O. Barber, an otoneurologist, and Charles W. Stockwell, a psychologist. The book described the anatomy and physiology of the vestibular system and the technique and interpretation for the electronystagmographic (ENG) examination. Additionally, the authors addressed report writing and supplied illustrative cases. All of this was covered exceedingly well in a concise 200 pages.

Since that time, the assessment of the vestibular system has broadened into the assessment of "balance function." The contemporary assessment includes measures of (a) ocular motility (ENG/VNG), (b) the integrity of the semicircular canal mediated vestibulo-ocular reflex (VOR) arc (ENG/VNG, sinusoidal harmonic acceleration testing), (c) the integrity of the saccule- and utricle-mediated VOR (vestibular-evoked myogenic potential and off-axis rotational testing), (d) evaluation of the vestibulospinal pathways [computerized dynamic posturography (CDP)], and (e) an assessment of multisensory integration of the three interdependent senses underlying balance (i.e., vision, somesthesia, and vestibular system function).

Most training programs for entry-level audiologist professionals have included two courses in their curriculum covering the assessment and management of balance disorders. In fact, it would be possible to create a curriculum of "vestibular sciences" courses that would represent analogs of the current graduate-level audiology courses. The addition of newer tests has resulted in a redefining of the relative importance of individual measures in the context of the comprehensive balance function test.

The purpose of this book is to provide the reader with a unitary source for protocols and procedures required for doing an ENG/VNG examination. The book is written for the graduate student or practicing clinician. In other words, the book is written from the perspective of a clinician with the intent of providing a text that can be used in the clinical environment. The first few chapters review the relevant anatomy and physiology of the vestibular and oculomotor systems. This is a basic review that is intended to provide a framework for understanding how impairments in these two systems can influence results and interpretation. The subsequent chapters focus on reviewing basic testing procedures and practical clinical matters. Incorporated into those chapters are the advances that have occurred over the past few decades in the assessment of dizziness and vertigo. For example, numerous studies have emerged in the areas of positioning testing and oculomotor assessment. Incorporated into this text are numerous case studies that the author has accumulated over the years and has found to be helpful in the training of students and colleagues. While this book serves as an introductory text, the reader should refer to the texts given in the references for a more extensive analysis.

Acknowledgments

I thank Gary Jacobson for his invaluable encouragement and help with editing, Barb Jacobson for her careful review of the manuscript, and Kamran Barin for his thoughtful suggestions and support. I also acknowledge my colleagues at the Vanderbilt Balance Disorders Clinic for providing cases and editing as well as support during this project. I especially thank my wife, Heather, for her love and patience, my son, Declan, who is always there to get me up in the morning, and my daughter, Molly, who knows how to keep me laughing.

1

Neural Control of Eye Movements

INTRODUCTION

One of the ways that an examiner can obtain information about a patient who complains of dizziness is to observe the patient's eye movements in response to different stimuli. In some instances, the observation of the eyes can be more sensitive than magnetic resonance imaging in localizing and identifying impairments that can result in balance disturbances. An examiner who is knowledgeable about the neurology of eye movements is afforded the ability to distinguish between impairments involving the central nervous system and the peripheral vestibular system.

HIERARCHY OF THE OCULOMOTOR SYSTEM

The neural control of human eye movements is organized in such a way as to allow an individual to explore their world in an effective way. When an object of visual interest is identified, three factors must be in play in order to observe it in detail (Schor, 2003): first, where the target is located; second, whether the target is moving or stationary; and third, whether the observer is moving or

stationary. Each of these considerations must be taken into account because of the physiological limitations of the retina. The retina is composed of two types of photoreceptor cells known as rods and cones. Cones are concentrated primarily in and around the fovea making it the part of the eye that has the highest spatial sensitivity and the part responsible for visual acuity (Figure 1–1). In this regard, when an observer wants to see a visual target with any detail, the oculomotor system (OMS) must align the two foveae so that the target falls

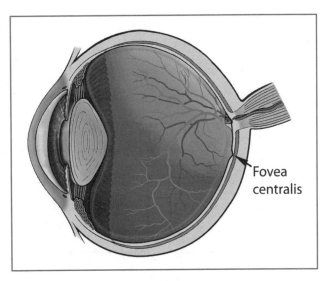

Fovea
centralis

FIGURE 1–1. A diagram of the eye illustrates the location of the fovea.

on them. A single type of eye movement is inadequate to keep targets of interest on the foveae in all situations and is the reason why multiple eye movement systems exist. Depending on the task required to observe a target, different eye movement systems with separate and independent neural pathways are recruited. Each of these systems employ different brain structures to process the information about the target, which ultimately converges in the "final common pathway."

Physiologists have organized the OMS into a hierarchy where each component has a different level of processing. Many authors organize the OMS into three components: (1) motor system, (2) premotor system, and (3) type of eye movement system. The motor system (i.e., the part of the system directly involved with movement of the eyes) moves the eye in the orbit and consists of the oculomotor nerves and the extraocular eye muscles. The premotor system organizes the neural input coming from higher centers (e.g., cerebral cortex and midbrain) and relays these commands to the motor system. The premotor system is located in the brainstem. Together, the motor and premotor systems comprise what has been termed the "final common pathway." Four primary control systems provide input to the final common pathway; these include the saccade, pursuit, optokinetic, and vestibular systems (Figure 1–2).

These systems all work together to enable an observer to clearly perceive objects of interest and explore the surrounding environment. First, the saccade system enables an observer to quickly bring a visual target identified in the peripheral field of vision system onto the fovea. The pursuit system is recruited when a target is moving slowly and the observer wishes to track it. The optokinetic and vestibular systems work together to keep the fovea centered on a target when the head is moving. The following section discusses the actions and neural generators of each of these functional classes of eye movements.

THE "FINAL COMMON PATHWAY" OF THE OCULOMOTOR SYSTEM

Sherrington (1947) described the final common pathway component of the OMS as being comprised of the ocular motor nerves and the extraocular muscles (EOMs). The EOMs are housed within

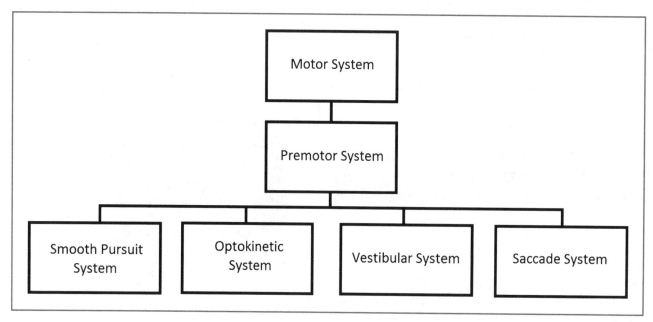

FIGURE 1–2. Primary control systems for the generation of eye movements. (Adapted from Barber & Stockwell, 1976)

the bone of the orbit. There are six EOMs that control the movement of each eye; these include the medial rectus, lateral rectus, superior rectus, inferior rectus, superior oblique, and inferior oblique (Figure 1–3). For each eye, these six muscles each have an opposing counterpart comprising three pairs. Each muscle in a pair moves the eye in the same plane but in the opposite

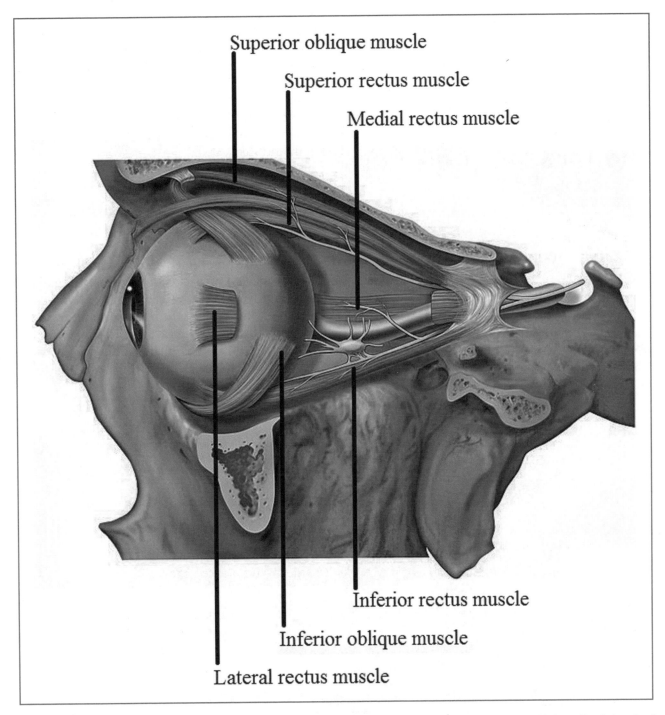

Superior oblique muscle

Superior rectus muscle

Medial rectus muscle

Inferior rectus muscle

Inferior oblique muscle

Lateral rectus muscle

FIGURE 1–3. The six extraocular muscles of the eye. (Courtesy of Patrick Lynch, Yale University School of Medicine)

direction (Figure 1–4). The eye can be moved in the horizontal plane (back and forth) and the vertical plane (up and down). A third type of movement is torsional. This is a rotation of the eye around the line of sight (an imaginary line that connects the eye with the target). The pairs are the medial rectus and lateral rectus, superior rectus and inferior rectus, and the superior and inferior oblique. If the eye is to be moved, the opposing counterpart (i.e., antagonist muscle) must be relaxed and the muscle pulling the eye in the direction of interest (i.e., agonist muscle) must be contracted. This type of action of the EOMs allows movement of the eye in three directional planes: horizontal, vertical, and torsional (Table 1–1). In the real world, the majority of eye movements are complex requiring various levels of activation and inhibition of all the EOMs. A comprehensive overview of this topic is given by Leigh and Zee (2006).

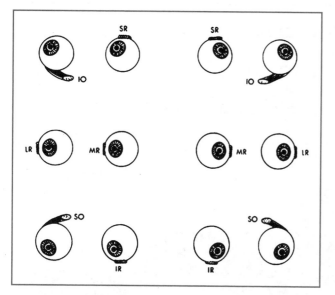

FIGURE 1–4. The different gaze positions and the primary agonist muscles that move the eye into position. **MR** medial rectus; **LR** lateral rectus; **SR** superior rectus; **IR** inferior rectus; **SO** superior oblique; **IO** inferior oblique. (From Barber & Stockwell, 1976)

Cranial Nerves and Nuclei of the Oculomotor System

The EOMs are innervated by oculomotor neurons (OMNs) located on each side of the midline of the brain (Figure 1–5). These cranial nuclei receive eye movement information from the premotor center and relay it through projections to innervate the EOMs. The cell bodies of these nerves form the three oculomotor nuclei: the third nucleus (oculomotor), the fourth nucleus (trochlear), and the

Table 1–1. Primary and Secondary Eye Movements Controlled by Extraocular Muscle

Extraocular Muscle	Primary Action	Secondary Action
Medial rectus	Moves eye inward	
Lateral rectus	Moves eye outward	
Superior rectus	Moves eye upward	Rotates top of eye toward nose
Inferior rectus	Moves eye downward	Rotates top of eye away from nose
Superior oblique	Rotates top of eye toward nose	Moves eye downward
Inferior oblique	Rotates top of eye away from nose	Moves eye upward

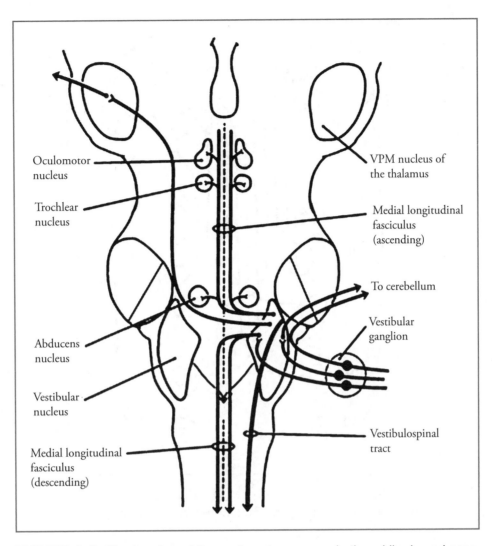

FIGURE 1–5. The location of the oculomotor neurons in the midbrain and pons. (From Fife, 2009)

sixth nucleus (abducens nucleus). The oculomotor nuclei are located in the midbrain near the floor of the third ventricle and innervate the ipsilateral medial rectus, inferior rectus, inferior oblique, and contralateral superior rectus. In addition, the third nucleus projects motor neurons to the iris sphincter and ciliary muscles of the eyes. The trochlear nuclei are found near the dorsal surface of the midbrain ventral and lateral to the aqueduct of Sylvius and innervate the contralateral superior oblique (Leigh & Zee, 2006). The abducens nuclei are located in the dorsal pons on the floor of the fourth ventricle and project to the ipsilateral lat-

eral rectus muscles. Figure 1–6 and Table 1–2 provide a summary of the EOMs and their respective innervation by the OMNs.

The OMNs control the velocity and position of the eye by continually adjusting the neural input to the EOMs. Constant neural activity is fed to the EOMs by the premotor system keeping them in a constant state of contraction which holds the eye steady in the orbit. In instances where the eye must be moved in a certain direction, motor neurons connected to the agonist muscles increase their neural drive to the agonist muscle (contracting it) while simultaneously decreasing their firing

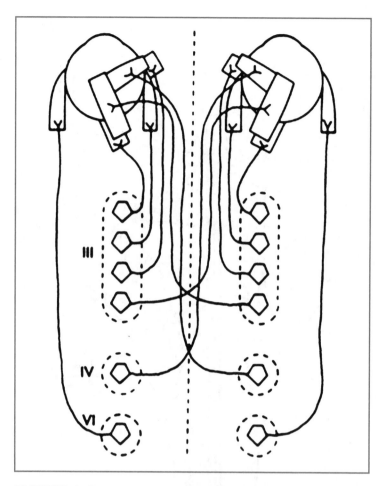

FIGURE 1–6. The extraocular muscles and their innervation by the oculomotor neurons. (From Barber & Stockwell, 1976)

Table 1–2. Cranial Nerve Innervation of Extraocular Muscles

Extraocular Muscle	Cranial Nerve Innervation
Medial rectus	Cranial nerve III (oculomotor)
Lateral rectus	Cranial nerve VI (abducens)
Superior rectus	Cranial nerve III (oculomotor)
Inferior rectus	Cranial nerve III (oculomotor)
Superior oblique	Cranial nerve IV (trochlear)
Inferior oblique	Cranial nerve III (oculomotor)

rate to the antagonist muscles and relaxing the opposing muscle.

Figure 1–7 shows how the neural drive from the OMNs moves the eye in the horizontal plane. In this illustration, the observer has detected a target that is 30° to the right, yet the eyes are oriented forward. In order to move the eye to the right, the EOMs responsible for moving the eye right in

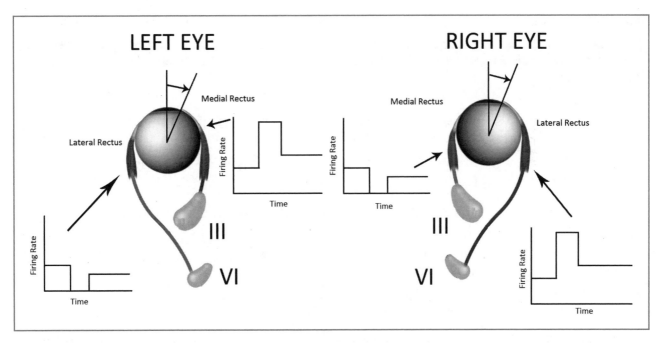

FIGURE 1–7. The relationship between changes in firing rate in the oculomotor neurons and the change in eye position for a rightward eye movement. (Adapted from Barber & Stockwell, 1976)

the horizontal plane must be contracted and their antagonists must be relaxed. The primary agonist muscles for this rightward movement of the eyes are the right lateral rectus and left medial rectus. In order to contract the lateral rectus and medial rectus, the abducens and oculomotor neurons increase their firing rates, respectively. The antagonist muscles are the left lateral rectus and right medial rectus, and the respective abducens and oculomotor neurons decrease their firing rate to these muscles causing them to relax and allow the eyeball to be moved to the right.

PREMOTOR SYSTEM

The human premotor oculomotor network involves a complex set of neural circuits that coordinate the generation of saccades, smooth pursuit, the vestibulo-ocular reflex (VOR), optokinetic nystagmus, VOR fixation, and gaze-holding (Leigh & Zee, 2006). This system receives neural input regarding the initiation, velocity, and accuracy of

slow and rapid eye movements from higher centers (e.g., cortex and midbrain) and organizes it into a neural signal that is sent to the motor system through direct and indirect projections. The premotor system has been described as being located in the brainstem tegmentum, and its role in eye movements is to provide the appropriate neural drive to the three oculomotor brainstem nuclei (i.e., oculomotor, trochlear, and abducens nuclei) (Barber & Stockwell, 1980). To completely describe the human premotor system is beyond the scope of this book; however, an extensive review of this system is given by Glaser (1991). An overview of the primary premotor structures, their functions, and associated eye movements are summarized in Table 1–3.

SACCADE SYSTEM

When a target is detected on the edge of the visual field, the OMS can quickly move the eye and place the image of interest on the fovea. This type of eye

Table 1–3. Overview of the Primary Premotor Structures, Their Functions, and Associated Eye Movements.

Premotor Structure	Function	Associated Eye Movement
Medial longitudinal fasiculus	Central conduit to the motor nuclei for coordinated and synchronized eye movements	Involved in all classes of eye movements
Superior colliculus	Generates quick eye movements for orienting to visual or auditory stimuli	Saccades
Superior and lateral vestibular nuclei	Plays a major role in the generation of the VOR and optokinetic nystagmus	VOR and optokinetic
Lateral vestibular nucleus	Fixes images with head stable and environment moving	Optokinetic
Pontine excitatory burst neurons	Generates ballistic eye movements for acquisition of a visual target	Saccade
Medial vestibular nucleus	Stabilizes images during head movement and stabilizes environment	VOR
Repositus hypoglossal (PPH)	Holds a target on the fovea	Together with the MVN it participates in horizontal gaze-holding

VOR vestibulo-ocular reflex; *MVN* medial vestibular nuclei

movement is known as a saccade and is the type of eye movement we use to shift our gaze to interesting targets and explore our visual environment (Robinson, 1964). The saccadic control system is responsible for generating extremely fast and accurate conjugate eye movements that place the foveae in new positions. The saccade is the fastest type of eye movement and its speed is dependent on the distance the eye must travel to acquire the target (faster for objects far away and slower for objects that are close). Saccades can be either reflexive or voluntary and occur in the absence of a visual stimulus (i.e., in the dark or with vision denied).

The calculation by the nervous system of what the amplitude of a voluntary saccade needs to be (i.e., how big the saccade has to be to acquire the target) involves what has been termed "retinal positional error" (RPE) (Heywood & Churcher, 1981). RPE describes the disparity between where the target is in space compared with where the retina is. A more specific way of describing this may be "foveae positional error" because it is the fovea that must be aligned with the target. When the target is identified, the entire process (i.e., premotor and motor contributions) of saccade generation takes, on average, less than 350 ms. The latency (i.e., how long before the eye begins to move) averages approximately 200–250 ms and most saccades last less than 100 ms (Rucker, 2010). As previously stated, the saccade system is capable of moving the eye extremely fast. This type of eye movement can range from approximately 100 to 800° per second. During this eye movement the observer is essentially "blind" because the retina is incapable of resolving images when the eye is moving at speeds this high.

Neural Mechanism

In order to accomplish this precise ballistic eye movement the system makes use of cortical, brainstem, and cerebellar circuitry (i.e., the neural integrator) to calculate where the fovea of the retina should go in order to fixate on an object of interest. A saccadic eye movement consists of three stages (Figure 1–8). First, the target must be

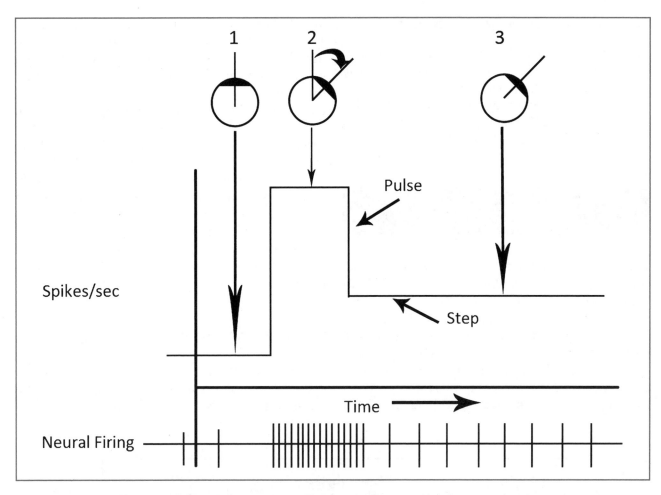

FIGURE 1–8. Relationship between the discharge rate and eye movement. *1* Eye is in primary position; *2* eye is quickly moved to the right; *3* eye is maintained in deviated position. (Adapted from Leigh & Zee, 2006)

identified and its location calculated. The decision to initiate a saccade is made by the higher centers (e.g., parietal cortex and frontal eye fields) that send converging information to a visuomotor integration center called the superior colliculus (SC) located on the dorsal aspect of the midbrain (Leigh & Zee, 2006). The SC relays the commands it receives from the higher centers to brainstem interneurons that code the required velocity and position coordinates to drive the motor neurons that move the eye from point "A" to point "B" (Figure 1–9). This is often referred to as the "pulse." The "pulse" generator has been localized to a brainstem center termed the paramedian pontine reticular formation. The second stage consists of a continued neural discharge that holds the eyes on the target, and this is known as the "step" response (see Figure 1–9). The "step" generator is

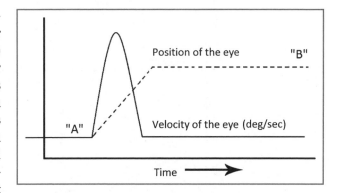

FIGURE 1–9. Relationship between the velocity of the eye and the position of the eye during a saccadic eye movement.

distributed throughout the brainstem and cerebellum. Together this neural process is known as the "pulse-step" (Sylvestre & Cullen, 1999).

Summary: Saccade Eye Movement

The purpose of saccade eye movement is to shift the gaze quickly from one target to another. The stimulus is a small or medium-size object not in the line of sight. Eye motion is rapid and conjugate. Latency is 200 ms. A recording of a random saccade test is shown in Figure 1–10.

PURSUIT SYSTEM

The pursuit system is a voluntary oculomotor control system that enables an observer to hold the foveae on a target that is moving slowly (<30° per second). The primary purpose of this system is to keep images stabilized on the fovea when the target is moving and the head is stable. Typically, a target is initially acquired quickly using the saccade system. If the target of interest is moving, the pursuit system is engaged to hold the visual target stable on the retina. The way the pursuit system holds the target on the retina is by continually sampling where the target is in relation to the fovea and adjusting for the amount that the target "slips" off the retina. The pursuit system is limited with regard to how fast it can track a target. When target velocities exceed 60° per second, the pursuit system is no longer able to match the eye velocity to the target velocity and the target is no longer maintained on the fovea. In this case the target must be reacquired using the saccade system. Interestingly, the pursuit system seems to be driven almost entirely by a moving visual stimulus. While one can produce saccades in the absence of visual stimuli, this is not true for pursuit.

Neural Mechanism

Smooth tracking of eye movements is accomplished using cortical, cerebellar, and brainstem centers. In order to track a visual target, a series

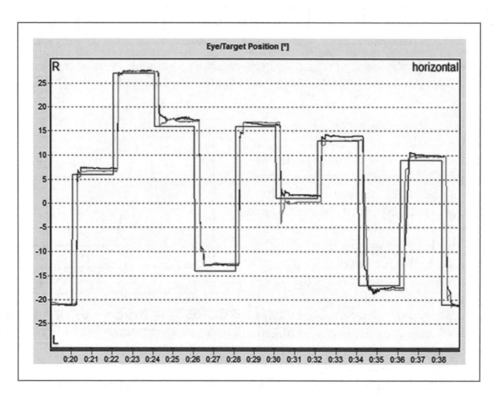

FIGURE 1–10. A recording of a normal random saccade paradigm and the associated eye movements (Interacoustics version; Interacoustics, Assens, Denmark)

of events must be accomplished which involve processing by each of the aforementioned centers. First, motion-sensitive cells in the fovea detect that an object is moving and they send signals about target velocity and direction to the visual cortex (e.g., parietal-occipital visual-association areas). From the visual cortex the information is relayed to motion-sensitive areas in the superior temporal sulcus (i.e., middle temporal (MT) area and medial superior temporal (MST) area) that in turn calculate the velocity of the target and distribute the updated information to the premotor systems (i.e., cerebellum, vestibular nucleus, and paramedian pontine reticular formation). The premotor system relays the processed information to the final common pathway (i.e., oculomotor nuclei and extraocular muscles) where the velocity of the eye is matched to the velocity of the object of interest.

Summary: Pursuit Eye Movement

The purpose of pursuit eye movement is to stabilize a moving image on the fovea. The stimulus is a small or medium-size object that is moving. Eye motion is slow, smooth, and conjugate. Latency is 100 ms. A recording of a pursuit test is shown in Figure 1–11.

GAZE-HOLDING: THE "NEURAL INTEGRATOR"

Gaze-holding describes the function of holding the foveae motionless on a target in the primary position or eccentric (deviated) position. When gaze is directed away from midline, the brain must program a tonic neural command of sufficient size to cause sustained contraction of the paired agonist extraocular muscles and a reciprocal command to decrease electrical tone delivered to the paired antagonist muscles. This is necessary to counteract the visuo-elastic restoring forces of the orbit that tend to pull back the eye to the primary position. This eye-position signal is generated by a gaze-holding network [i.e., the neural integrator (NI)].

Neural Mechanism

The NI is a distributed function (i.e., distributed among several structures in the brainstem) and is highly dependent on an intact vestibulocerebellum (flocculus and paraflocculus) (Leigh & Zee, 2006). When patients with impairments in the NI are asked to hold their eyes on a target in an eccentric

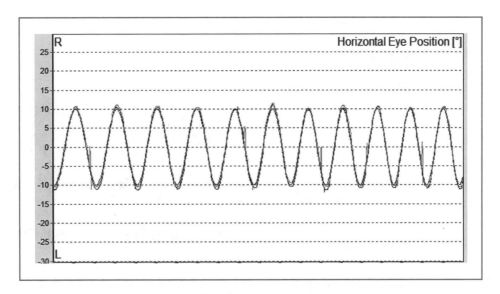

FIGURE 1–11. A recording of the eye movements in response to a pursuit stimulus (Interacoustics version; Interacoustics, Assens, Denmark)

position, they often demonstrate a slow drift of their eyes off the target followed by a quick corrective saccade of the eye back onto the target (Figure 1–12). When gazing at a target in an eccentric position, the NI is continuously updating the neural command to extraocular muscles to ensure that the eyes stay on the target; however, impairment in this gaze-holding system results in a reduced step response and thus a centripetal drift of the eyes off the target. A corrective saccade directed away from the primary position is generated by the OMS to reacquire the target. This phenomenon has been termed gaze-evoked nystagmus, and it manifests as a jerk nystagmus that is characterized by a low amplitude and high frequency.

Summary: Gaze Eye Movement

The purpose of gaze eye movement is to stabilize an image on the fovea that is not in the line of sight. The stimulus is a small or medium-size object that is stationary. Eye motion is conjugate. Latency is not applicable.

OPTOKINETIC SYSTEM

The optokinetic (OKN) system is a reflexive functional class of eye movement that works in concert with the vestibular system to stabilize a moving visual environment on the retina when the head is stationary. This subsystem generates a response that is complementary to the one that is provided by the labyrinths (Leigh & Zee, 2006). Together, the responses from the OKN system and the vestibular system generate a slow compensatory eye movement that is proportional to the velocity of the head movement. When the head velocity is slow, the compensatory input is driven primarily by the OKN system; however, when the head is moved at a frequency above approximately 1 Hz, the input is provided primarily by the peripheral vestibular system. Stimuli moving to the right are slowly followed by both eyes. Once the eyes reach a certain position in the orbit, they are quickly reset in the opposite direction at which point the

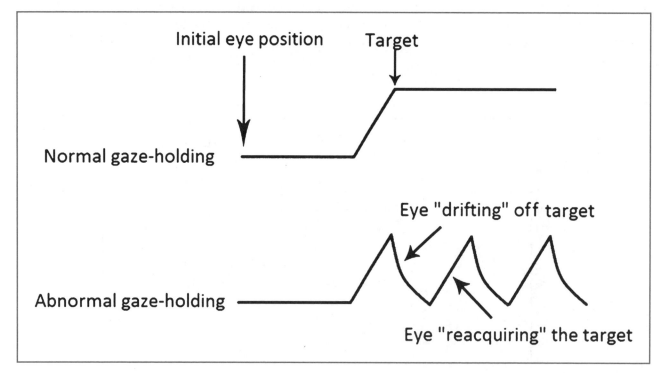

FIGURE 1–12. A comparison of normal gaze-holding and abnormal gaze-holding and the associated eye movement.

stimuli are reacquired and tracked again. This slow tracking movement (which has the same velocity as the head movement) followed by the quick resetting of the eye in the opposite direction has been termed optokinetic nystagmus (Figure 1–13).

Neural Mechanism

In order to generate compensatory eye movements that are appropriate for observing the moving visual stimulus, the OKN system processes the visual input using two different pathways. OKN eye movement is initiated at the retina, which contains ganglionic cells that respond exclusively to motion in certain directions and orientations.

Motion-generated signals sent from the retina pass through the optic nerve at which point the signal diverges and inputs are sent to the cortex (via lateral geniculate nucleus) and brainstem.

The brainstem pathway receives the OKN signals from the optic nerve. At a certain point they decussate at the optic chiasm and are projected to specialized nuclei in the brainstem [i.e., nucleus of the optic tract (NOT)] that code motion. Specifically, the NOT is composed of cells with receptive fields sensitive to moving stimuli. Once the NOT has received the input from the contralateral eyes, it relays the signals to the vestibular nuclei. The vestibular nuclei project this electrical code to the OMNs that drive eye movement to track the moving stimulus. The

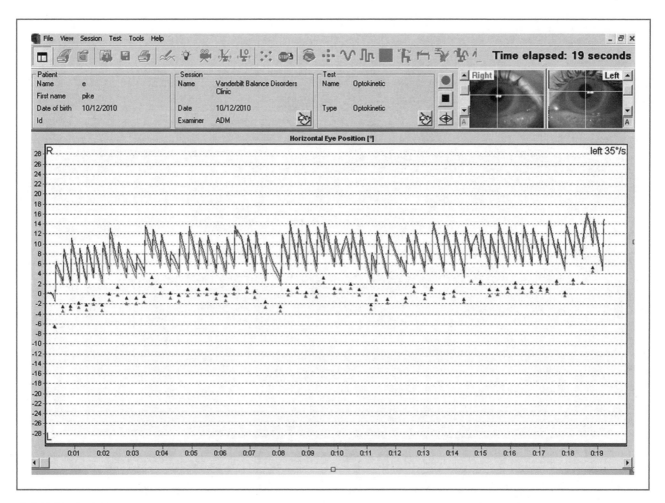

FIGURE 1–13. A recording of the eye movements in response to a full-field optokinetic stimulus consisting of stripes (Interacoustics version; Interacoustics, Assens, Denmark)

cortical pathway receives and processes the target information, which is routed via the lateral geniculate nucleus to the MST, where information regarding ipsilateral motion is coded. This visual input, which has been processed by the cortex, is relayed to the NOT and then to the premotor system to move the eye accordingly.

Summary: OKN Eye Movement

The purpose of OKN eye movement is to stabilize an image of interest during sustained head movements. The stimulus is a steady-moving full-field visual environment. Eye motion is rapid and slow alternating eye movements (nystagmus). Latency is 75 ms.

2

Anatomy and Physiology of the Vestibular System

INTRODUCTION

The vestibular system is composed of a set of five electrical generators, or end organs, on each side that accomplish three primary tasks. First, it acts to provide information to the central nervous system for controlling skeletal muscle tone for adjusting posture. Second, it works to stabilize the visual environment when the visual surrounding is moving or the observer is moving. Third, it provides the central nervous system with spatial information regarding linear and angular movements. The peripheral vestibular system is an elegant network of membranous sacs (i.e., membranous labyrinth) located in the petrous portion of the temporal bone within a bony labyrinth (Figure 2–1). The membranous labyrinth is suspended within the bony labyrinth by connective tissue and is surrounded by perilymph that has an ionic composition that is high in Na+ and low in K+ (Figure 2–2). The five organs that make up the vestibular apparatus are the three semicircular canals (i.e., horizontal, anterior, and posterior) and two otolith organs (i.e., utricle and saccule). Each canal has an enlarged end called an ampulla that contains a sensory organ. The canals are filled with endolymph, which is a substance that is high in K+ and low in Na+. The otoliths organs act as inertial accelerometers and each have a sensory organ known as the maculae. Anatomically, the semicircular canals (SCCs) and otolith organs are, at the same time, both similar and different. Each organ has a mass that is connected to stereocilia that project from the tops of specialized hair cells. It is the effect of inertia during acceleration or deceleration on the mass that results in a movement of the cilia and electrical transduction at the base of the hair cells (Figure 2–3).

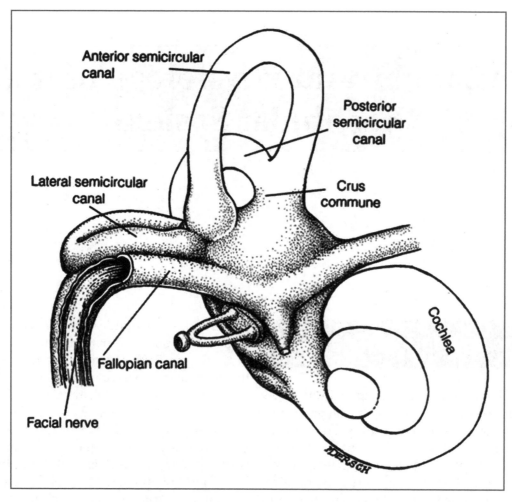

FIGURE 2–1. The anatomy of the bony labyrinth. (Illustration by Mary Dersch from Pender, 1992, with permission of Daniel Pender)

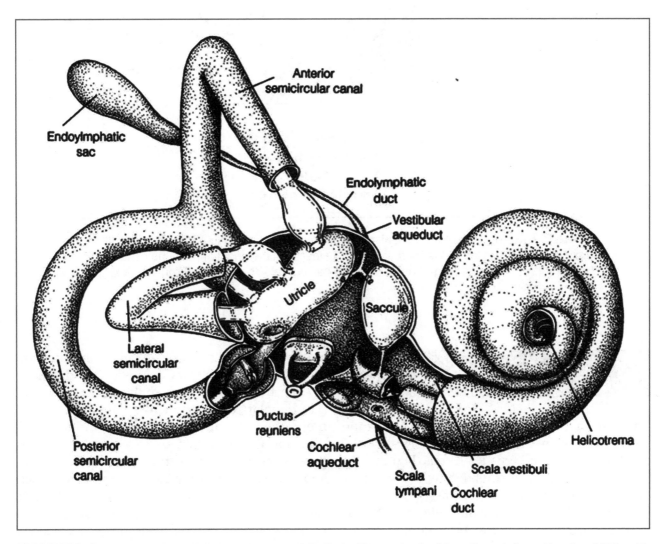

FIGURE 2–2. The anatomy of the membranous labyrinth. (Illustration by Mary Dersch from Pender, 1992, with permission of Daniel Pender)

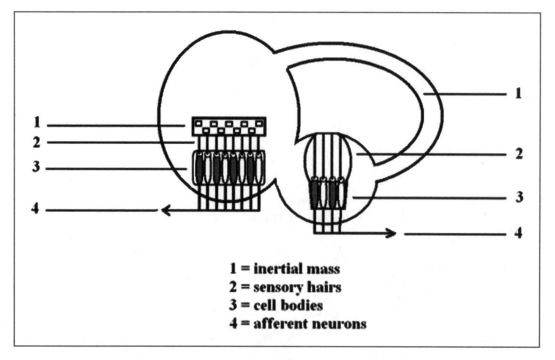

FIGURE 2–3. The receptor mechanisms of the semicircular canals (SCCs) and otolith system. The stimulus of the SCCs is provided by the inertia of the endolymph in the canal system. The stimulus of the otolith organs is provided by the inertia of the otoliths. (From Musiek, Baran, Shinn, & Jones, 2012)

VESTIBULAR HAIR CELLS

There are two primary types of hair cells in the vestibular system; these are the cylindrical type II and the flask-shaped type I hair cells (Figure 2–4). Type I hair cells are surrounded by a large calyx at the base of the cell. In contrast to the type I cells, type II hair cells have multiple nerve terminals connecting at the base. In the cupula, type I hair cells are centered on the top of the cristae in the SCCs and near the striola on the utricle and saccule. Type II hair cells are focused around the sides of the crista and on the lateral edges of the otoliths organs. Both types of hair cells have stereocilia that progressively increase in height. The stereocilia form a gradient from shortest to tallest terminating on a single longer and thicker kinocilium. The stimulus for the hair cells in the vestibular system is mechanical force. A parallel force applied to the top of the stereocilia in the direction of the kinocilium allows the K+ rich endolymph to enter the cell and increase the resting potential (i.e., depolarize it) and increase the firing rate in the nerve. An equivalent force in the opposite direction (away from the kinocilium) decreases the resting potential of the cell (hyperpolarize) and decreases the firing rate in the nerve. When a force perpendicular (straight down) to the hair cells is applied, there is little or no change in the resting potential of the cells (Hudspeth & Corey, 1977; Hudspeth, 1982).

SEMICIRCULAR CANAL ANATOMY AND PHYSIOLOGY

The three SCCs are arranged orthogonally (at right angles) to each other enabling the system to detect the direction and amplitude of a head

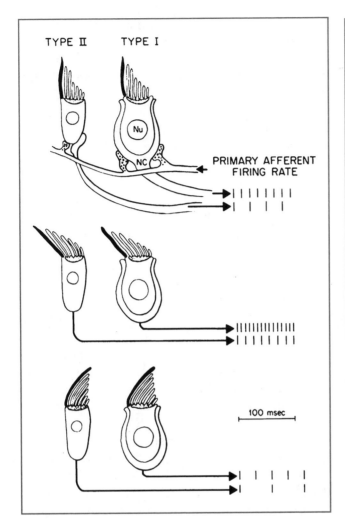

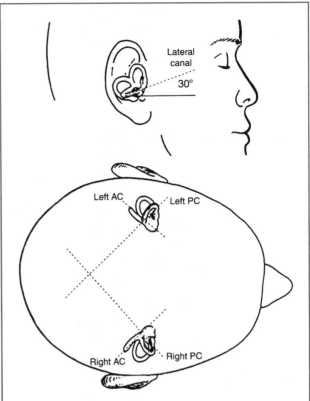

FIGURE 2–5. Spatial orientation of the SCCs. **AC** anterior canal; **PC** posterior canal. (From Eggers & Zee, 2010)

FIGURE 2–4. A representation of the firing of primary vestibular afferent neurons for different directions of deflection of type I and type II hair cells. (From Baloh, 1998b)

movement in any direction. The two vertical SCCs are oriented at 45° in the sagittal plane and the horizontal canals are tilted upward approximately 30°. Each SCC canal has a partner on the opposite side that is coplanar and detects movement in the same plane (Figure 2–5). When one member of the pair is stimulated (i.e., excited) by a head movement in the plane of stimulation for that canal, the partner is inhibited. For instance, when the head is moved quickly to the right in the horizontal plane, the right horizontal SCC is excited and its counterpart the left horizontal SCC is inhibited. The pair-

ings for the vertical canals are the right anterior and left posterior (RALP) and the left anterior and right posterior (LARP) canals.

Each SCC has an enlarged end called the ampulla (Lysakowski, 2005). The ampulla houses each canal's sensory epithelium (i.e., crista ampullaris). The crista ampullaris is shaped like a dome and is composed of several parts. One component of the crista ampullaris is the cupula. The cupula is a gelatinous mass that extends from the base of the ampulla to the roof and effectively seals off the two sides of the ampulla (Figure 2–6) (McLaren & Hillman, 1979). Embedded in the base of the cupula are the stereocilia of the type I and type II receptor hair cells. The approximately 7,000 hair cells in each of the crista are polarized in the same direction (Berthoz, 1996). In this regard, a deflection of the hair cell bundle toward the kinocilium results in an increase in firing rate of the afferent fibers connected to the hair cell. Deflection of the stereocilia bundle away from the kinocilium

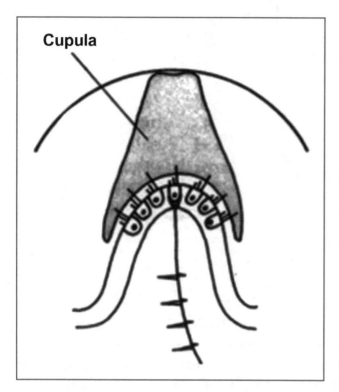

FIGURE 2–6. The crista ampullaris is shown. (Illustration by Mary Dersch from Pender, 1992, with permission of Daniel Pender)

results in a decrease in neural afferent firing rate (Figure 2–7). The stereocilia in the vertical canals (anterior and posterior) are polarized toward the canal side of the ampulla. The stereocilia in the horizontal canals are oriented toward the utricular side of the ampulla. This arrangement creates a difference in the directional sensitivity of the vertical and horizontal canals (Figure 2–8). In the horizontal canals, movement of endolymph toward the ampulla (ampullopetal) generates an increase in firing rate in the nerve while in the vertical canals the opposite is true (endolymph flow toward the ampulla results in a decrease firing rate in the nerve). The distribution of the hair cells in the cristae is complex (Brichta & Goldberg, 1996). Type I hair cells produce an irregular firing pattern and are found to be clustered in the center of the crista (Goldberg & Fernandez, 1971a, 1971b). Goldberg, Highstein, Moschovakis, and Fernandez (1987) suggest that this arrangement of the type I hair cells in the crista may be responsible for producing quick bursts of neural activity that adjust the head when the canals are stimulated. In contrast, type II neurons are found to be located on the periphery of the crista and have been suggested to be primarily responsible for driving the eye movement of the vestibuloocular reflex (VOR) (Goldberg et al., 1987). The cupula and the endolymph surrounding it have essentially the same

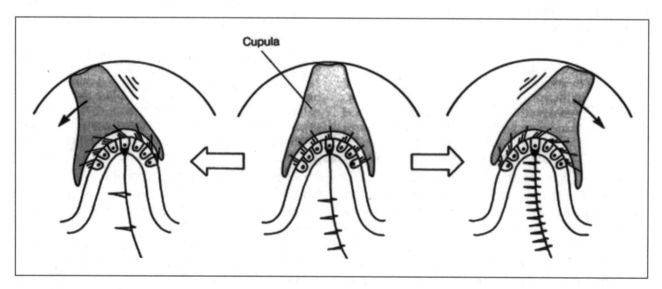

FIGURE 2–7. Cupular deflection in one direction results in an increase in firing in the nerve and a decrease in the opposite direction. (Illustration by Mary Dersch from Pender, 1992, with permission of Daniel Pender)

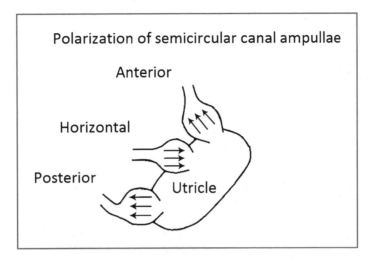

FIGURE 2–8. Polarization patterns of the hair cells in the SCCs. The *arrows* indicate the directions in which the stereocilia are oriented.

specific gravity making the cristae insensitive to gravity. When the head is still, the cupula is suspended in the endolymph in a neutrally buoyant position and the vestibular afferents fire at their tonic resting rate; however, when the head is moved in an angular fashion, the endolymph lags behind the canal walls. When this happens the cupula acts as a partition in the ampullar cavity and the endolymph presses on the cupula and bends it in the opposite direction of the head movement. When the hair cells embedded in the base of each of the cupula are deflected, ion channels in the tips of the stereocilia open or close (depending on the direction of the head movement) and allow more or less endolymph into the cell as compared with when the system is at rest. More endolymph entering the cell raises the resting potential and increases the amount of activation that occurs at the synapses between the cell and the nerve (increasing the firing rate in the nerve). This excitatory action is known as an ampullopetal response. Less endolymph entering the cell lowers the resting potential and decreases the activation of the synapses between the cell and the nerve (decreasing the firing rate in the nerve). This inhibitory action is termed an ampullofugal response. These changes in the vestibular nerve firing rate drive the compensatory eye movements of the VOR and are discussed later.

OTOLITH ORGAN ANATOMY AND PHYSIOLOGY

While the ENG/VNG examination does not assess the otolith organs, a basic understanding of them is necessary for any clinician assessing balance function. The two otolith organs are the saccule and utricle, and each has a sensory epithelium called a maculae. The utricular macule is oriented in the horizontal plane and lies near the anterior opening of the horizontal SCC. The macule of the saccule is oriented primarily in the vertical plane and is located on the medial wall of the vestibule inferior to the utricle (Figure 2–9). There are small (i.e., 5–7 µm) calcium carbonate crystals ($Ca(CO_3)$) referred to as "otoconia" that act as the mass in the utricle and the saccule (Figure 2–10) (Ross, Donovan, & Chee 1985). The crystals are dense compared with the surrounding endolymph and therefore have a higher specific gravity (i.e., they are heavier) (Money et al., 1971).

The macules are composed of several components that enable them to effectively transduce and code linear acceleration. First, the otoconia are embedded in a gelatinous matrix known as the otolithic membrane. The otolithic membrane of the utricle is loosely attached to the skull and it transduces head movement in primarily the

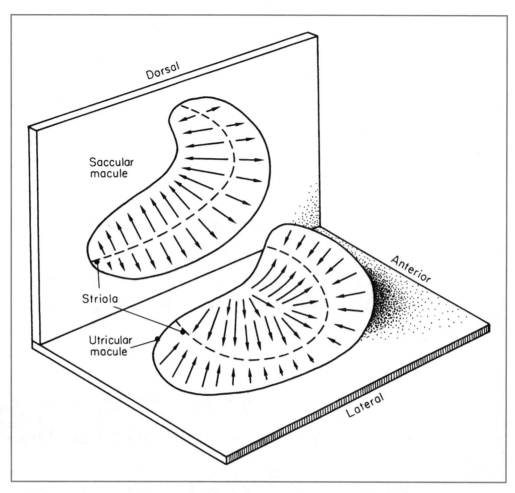

FIGURE 2–9. Orientation of the maculae of the utricle and saccule. The *arrows* indicate the direction in which the stereocilia are oriented. (From Baloh, 1998b)

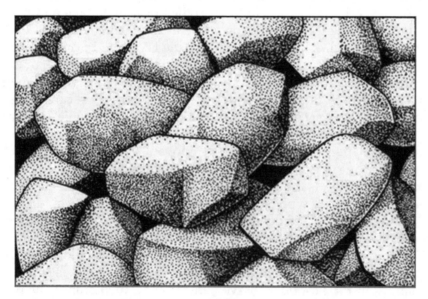

FIGURE 2–10. Otoconia is shown. (Illustration by Mary Dersch from Pender, 1992, with permission of Daniel Pender)

horizontal plane. The otolithic membrane of the saccule is more firmly attached and processes the constant pull of gravity as well as vertical head translations (Fettiplace & Fuchs, 1999). The cilia projecting from the hair cells in both maculae are embedded into the bottom of each otolithic membrane. In this way, the maculae act as bio-accelerometers that are sensitive to linear motion. Given that the otolithic membranes of the saccule and utricle are heavier than the endolymph, a shift or tilt of the head displaces them, so they align with the earth's vertical gravity vector (Fernández & Goldberg, 1976). Furthermore, when the head is translated quickly, the free-floating nature of the otolithic membranes causes them to lag behind resulting in a deflection of the hair cells in the direction opposite that of the head movement (Figure 2–11).

In contrast to the cristae, the polarization patterns of the hair cells in the maculae are more complex. Each macula has a line running through it which is composed of very small otoconia. This anatomical line is known as a striola and it acts to divide the maculae into two parts. In the saccular macula the hair cells are oriented in opposing directions around the striola. In the utricular macula, the hair cells are oriented toward the striola. This pattern of polarization enables an organism to sense linear head motion in nearly any direction.

The saccule has two systems that it employs to enhance its response sensitivity to tilt and linear acceleration. First, like the SCCs, commissural fibers exist between the two saccules. When saccular afferents are stimulated they receive ipsilateral excitation and contralateral inhibition via the commissural fibers; however, it has been reported that only 10% of second-order neurons excited by ipsilateral saccular afferent stimulation receive commissural inhibition (Uchino, 2001). This suggests that during linear acceleration (deceleration) the saccule is less dependent on the contralateral end organ to produce an electrical asymmetry (for detecting motion) than are SCCs. The second mechanism employed by the saccule to increase its sensitivity has been termed "cross-striolar inhibition" (Uchino, 2001). The mechanism of excitation and inhibition in the saccule is related to the geometric arrangement of the hair cells around the striola. When a linear acceleration occurs, some hair cells are depolarized while others on the side opposite the striola are hyperpolarized; thus, each saccule is independently capable of producing an electrical asymmetry necessary for the detection of motion. The majority of the vestibular neurons that are modulated by cross-striolar inhibition have axonal projections to the spinal cord (Sato, Ohkawa, Uchino, & Wilson, 1997); therefore, if one saccule is impaired by disease, information from the intact saccule will

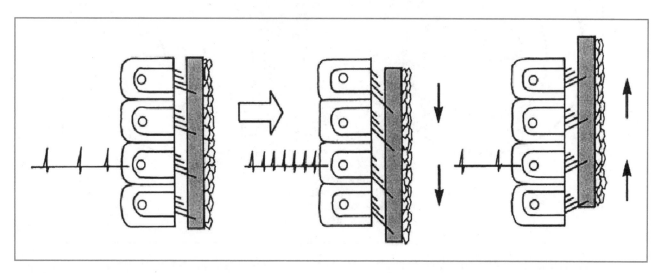

FIGURE 2–11. Mechanism of macule hair cell activation. (Illustration by Mary Dersch from Pender, 1992, with permission of Daniel Pender)

still be available to the central vestibular system to adjust posture and eye movements. The SCC system does not benefit from this redundancy and thus may help to explain why patients with canal impairments suffer poorer postural stability than their counterparts with unilaterally impaired saccules (McCaslin et al., 2007).

PRIMARY VESTIBULAR AFFERENT PROJECTIONS

Each of the end organs in the peripheral vestibular system sends their dendrites to the cell bodies located in Scarpas's ganglion (SG). SG is the origin of the two branches of the vestibular nerve that are located in the internal auditory canal. One division is termed the superior (anterior) vestibular nerve and it innervates the horizontal and anterior cristae, utricle, and a small portion of the saccule macule. The inferior (posterior) vestibular nerve innervates the posterior SCC and the inferior division of the saccule macule. The inferior and superior vestibular nerves run together as a bundle into the lateral medulla (Figure 2–12). The two vestibular branches of the vestibular nerve are composed of approximately 25,000 single nerve fibers that have a firing rate between 10 and 100 spikes/second (Ishiyama, Lopez, Ishiyama, & Tang, 2004; Ishiyama et al., 2005). According to Rasmussen (1940), the number of afferent nerve

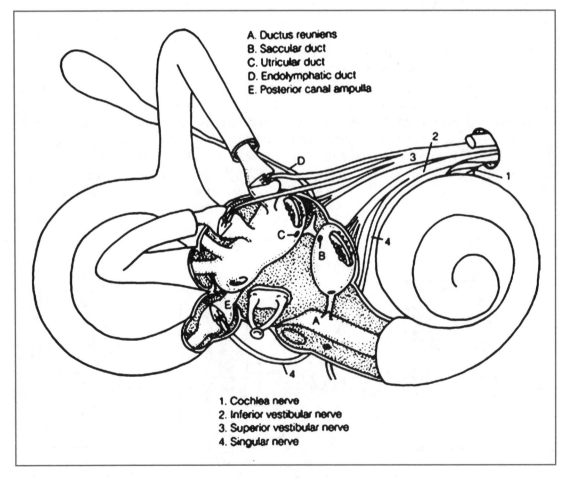

A. Ductus reuniens
B. Saccular duct
C. Utricular duct
D. Endolymphatic duct
E. Posterior canal ampulla

1. Cochlea nerve
2. Inferior vestibular nerve
3. Superior vestibular nerve
4. Singular nerve

FIGURE 2–12. Afferent nerve fibers from the vestibular receptors. (Illustration by Mary Dersch from Pender, 1992, with permission of Daniel Pender)

fibers is evenly distributed between the otolith organs and the SCCs. Type I hair cells located in the middle of the cristae are innervated by the largest-diameter nerve fibers while the smallest nerve fibers connect to type II hair cells in the lateral regions of the macules and cristae. The primary excitatory neurotransmitter of the vestibular afferents is glutamate (Straka, Biesdorf, & Dieringer, 2000).

Blood Supply to the Peripheral Vestibular System

The primary source of blood supply to the membranous labyrinth is the labyrinthine artery which, in most instances, originates from the antero-inferior cerebellar artery (Figure 2–13) (Mazzoni 1969). When the labyrinthine artery enters the temporal bone it feeds structures within the internal auditory canal. Upon entering the inner ear, the labyrinthine artery bifurcates into two divisions: the common cochlear artery and the anterior vestibular artery. The common cochlear artery further divides in the main cochlear artery and the posterior cochlear vestibular artery. The main cochlear artery irrigates the spiral ganglion. The posterior vestibular artery supplies the ampulla of the posterior canal and the inferior portion of the saccule. The anterior vestibular artery supplies the utricle, the ampulla of the horizontal and superior canals, and a small part of the saccule. The selective supply of the vestibular end organs by different arteries can lead to various patterns of pathology during quantitative testing.

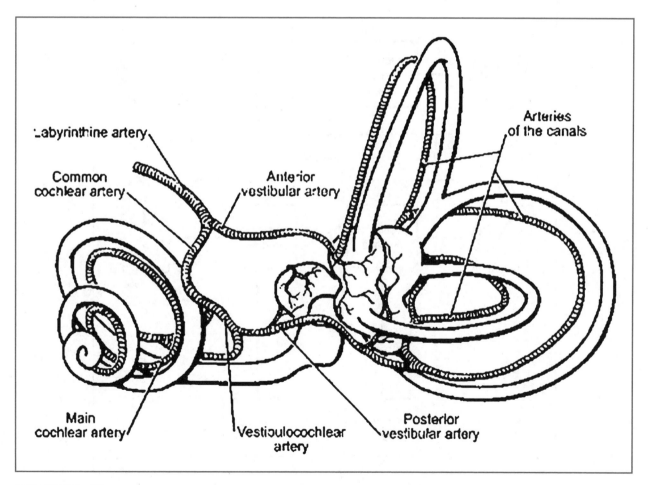

FIGURE 2–13. Arterial supply to the inner ear. (From Eggers & Zee, 2010)

ANATOMY OF THE CENTRAL VESTIBULAR SYSTEM

Primary vestibular afferents divide into an ascending and descending branch as they enter the brainstem and project to second-order neurons in the vestibular nuclei (VN) (i.e., the vestibular equivalent of the cochlear nuclei). The ascending branch terminates on cells in the cerebellum or rostral portion of the VN. The descending branch sends projections to the caudal portion of the VN. The VN are located on the floor of the fourth ventricle in the pons. There are four anatomical divisions of the VN (i.e., superior, medial, lateral, and inferior). The VN serve as the primary distribution center for neural activity generated by the peripheral vestibular system (Figure 2–14). The innervation of the VN by the peripheral vestibular system is extremely complex; however,

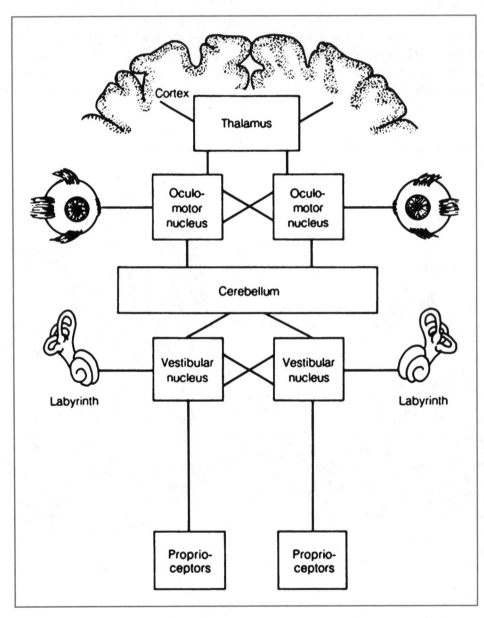

FIGURE 2–14. Connections between the peripheral and central vestibular systems. (Illustration by Mary Dersch from Pender, 1992, with permission of Daniel Pender)

the majority of the fibers coming from the canal system synapse on the medial and superior nuclei while the projections from the otolith organs terminate in the lateral and medial nuclei. The neural activity received by the VN from the canal and otolith organs is analyzed and then routed in different ways through a number of different systems depending on balance needs of the individual. For example, the eye movement pathway receives vestibular input from the VN in order to make adjustments to the eyeball in the orbit so that objects can be viewed clearly while the person is walking or running (VOR). The VN also receives direct neural input from the cerebellum (e.g., vermis and flocculonodular lobe) (Figure 2–15). The

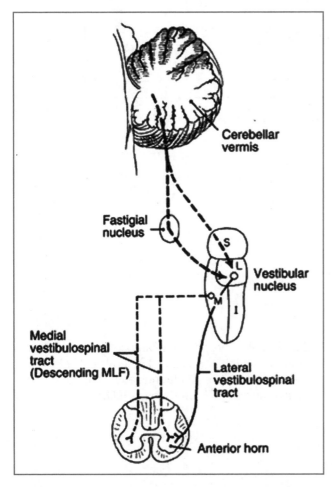

FIGURE 2–15. Vestibulocerebellar and vestibulospinal projections. **S** superior vestibular nucleus; **L** lateral vestibular nucleus; **M** medial vestibular nucleus; **I** inferior vestibular nucleus; **MLF** medial longitudinal fasciculus. (From Baloh, 1998b)

connections between the cerebellar structures and the VN are what make it possible for patients to recover function following impairment (i.e., improve the dynamic properties of the VOR and vestibulospinal reflex) to a single end organ (Ito, 1993). They also work to coordinate movements of the eyes and the head. Connections also exist between the VN and the descending spinal cord pathways (i.e., the lateral and medial vestibulospinal pathways, and the reticulospinal pathway) that are responsible for posture and gait. There are also strong connections between the VN, the reticular activating system, and the autonomic nervous system (Figure 2–16). These systems contribute to the secondary reactions, such as pallor, sweating, nausea, and vomiting, that occur when an individual suffers from a loss of function in one of the end organs. Finally, areas in the cortex indirectly receive input from the peripheral vestibular system by way of the brainstem. These cortical areas contribute to the perception of motion (Figure 2–17). The vestibulocortical pathway has been reported to include projections from the superior and lateral VN, the thalamus, and the parietal and temporal lobes of the cortex (Berthoz, 1996). It has been suggested that the functional aspect of the projections to the cortex is to bind vestibular, proprioceptive, and visual sensory input into one percept of spatial orientation (Baloh, 1998a).

Semicircular Canal and Ocular Pairings

The SCCs and eyes are linked through a series of pathways that extend from the peripheral vestibular system to the EOMs by way of the brainstem. Afferent projections from the ampullas of the canals project to the VN which then connect to the motorneurons of the EOMs. When the SCCs are accelerated in their plane of stimulation, the eyes are moved in approximately the same plane (Flouren's law). This phenomenon is facilitated by the fact that each EOM receives both excitatory and inhibitory input from the canal system (Ito et al., 1977). Furthermore, afferent input from each canal is sent to one muscle attached to the ipsilateral eye and one muscle attached to the contralateral eye. As described previously, each SCC canal

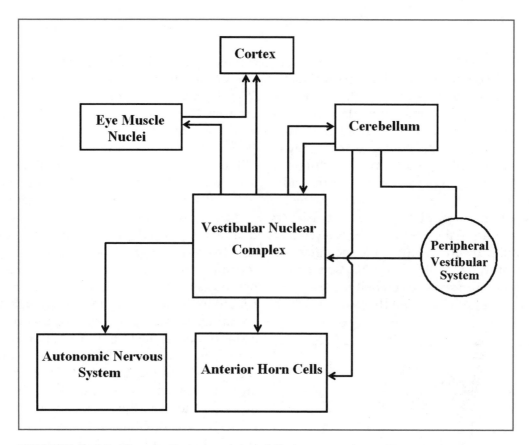

FIGURE 2–16. The vestibular nuclei and their connections. (From Musiek, Baran, Shinn, & Jones, 2012)

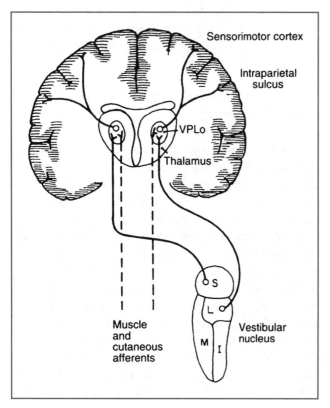

FIGURE 2–17. Vestibulothalamocortical pathways. **S** superior vestibular nucleus; **L** lateral vestibular nucleus; **M** medial vestibular nucleus; **I** inferior vestibular nucleus. (From Baloh, 1998b)

has a partner on the opposite side that is coplanar and detects movement in the same plane (e.g., RALP and LARP). In other words, any angular acceleration that increases neural firing rate in one canal also causes a corresponding decrease in the firing rate in its partner on the opposite side (Figure 2–18). This type of arrangement is known in engineering terms as a push-pull organization. Given that each canal sends projections to the opposing eye muscles of its partner, the eyes move in the opposite direction of the head movement. An example of how this system works would be when the head is moved in the RALP plane. In this case, when the head is moved in a manner that stimulates the anterior canal, there is an increase in neural activity routed to the ipsilateral superior rectus and contralateral inferior oblique, and muscle tone is increased (the muscles are contracted). Simultaneously, the left inferior canal is moved in such a way as to reduce the firing rate in the nerve (ampullofugally) and the ipsilateral inferior oblique and contralateral superior rectus are inhibited resulting in a decrease in muscle tone in these muscles. A summary of the excitatory and inhibitory connections from each canal is presented in Table 2–1. These slow reflexive movements of the eyes that occur with stimulation of the peripheral vestibular system during head movement are one component of the VOR.

The connections between the horizontal SCCs are of particular interest because these are the canals that are most commonly assessed during the ENG/VNG examination. The horizontal VOR is the primary reflex that is measured during the caloric portion of the ENG/VNG examination. It is a neural circuit that has an extremely short latency and is evoked with movement of the head or body. The purpose of the VOR is to enable clear vision in dynamic situations by moving the eyes in an equal and opposite direction of the head movement. This type of action keeps the fovea on the object of interest allowing for clear vision during dynamic situations. An example of this reflex in action is the ability of a person running on a treadmill to read a magazine or watch a monitor

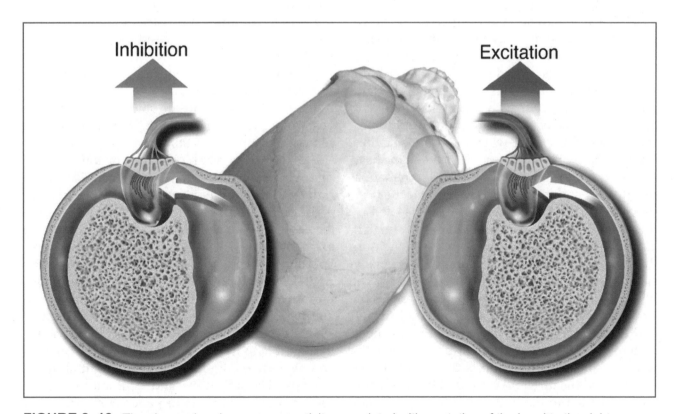

FIGURE 2–18. The change in primary nerve activity associated with a rotation of the head to the right.

Table 2–1. Summary of the Excitatory and Inhibitory Connections in Three Canals

Semicircular Canal	Extraocular Muscles Excited	Extraocular Muscles Inhibited
Posterior (inferior)	Ipsilateral (SO)	Ipsilateral (IO)
	Contralateral (IR)	Contralateral (SR)
Anterior (superior)	Ipsilateral (SR)	Ipsilateral (IR)
	Contralateral (IO)	Contralateral (SO)
Horizontal (lateral)	Ipsilateral (MR)	Ipsilateral (LR)
	Contralateral (LR)	Contralateral (MR)

Adapted from Barin (2009)

SO superior oblique; *IO* inferior oblique; *IR* inferior rectus; *SR* superior rectus; *MR* medial rectus; *LR* lateral rectus

at the same time. The horizontal VOR is shown in Figure 2–19.

When the head is stationary, the tonic firing rate in the primary vestibular afferents on both sides is essentially equal and the eyes do not move. It is angular acceleration and deceleration of the head that is the stimulus that activates the VOR. When an individual turns their head quickly to the right, the skull (and the membranous labyrinths) moves to the right; however, because of the inertial properties of endolymph it lags behind. A good explanation of this phenomenon is Newton's law of inertia: "An object at rest will remain at rest unless acted on by an unbalanced force." In the case of the VOR, when the head is stationary, the endolymph is not moving. When the head is moved, the endolymph is inclined to remain at rest due to inertia, and so it lags behind the head movement. Given that the ampulla is sealed by the cupula, the endolymph cannot pass through it. This causes a corresponding increase in pressure that occurs on one side of each cupula (opposite sides) causing them to bend. In the case of the head turn to the right, the right lateral canal is the leading ear for the head movement, and the left end organ is housed in the lagging ear. A head turn to the right causes endolymph to flow to the left and consequently deflects the cupula to the left (toward the utricle). Given that the stereocilia are embedded in the bottom of the cupula, they are also deflected. The deflection of the stereo-

cilia toward the utricle opens the ion channels in their tips and allows endolymph to flow into the cell. As endolymph enters the cell, the resting potential increases resulting in an increase in activity at the synaptic junction at the base of the cell increasing firing in the nerve. Conversely, the cupula in the left ear is deflected away from the utricle (inhibitory or utriculofugal) driving the firing rate in the left vestibular nerve below its tonic resting rate.

The changes in baseline firing rate in the superior vestibular nerves caused by the acceleration of the head to the right are routed to the medial vestibular nuclei (MVN). In the example presented, the superior vestibular nerve on the right side is firing at a rate higher than its tonic resting rate which increases the level of activity in the right MVN. A simultaneous decrease in firing rate occurs in the left MVN. The right MVN projects the increased level of neural activity to both ipsilateral and contralateral secondary vestibular neurons. Specifically, the right MVN sends projections to the right oculomotor nucleus (III) and sends decussating projections to the left abducens nucleus (VI). On the left side, a similar but opposite chain of events occurs. The left MVN relays the decrease in neural activity to the left oculomotor nucleus and also across the midline to the right abduces nucleus. The abducens and oculomotor nuclei send motor projections to the effector organs of the horizontal VOR (i.e., extraocular muscles).

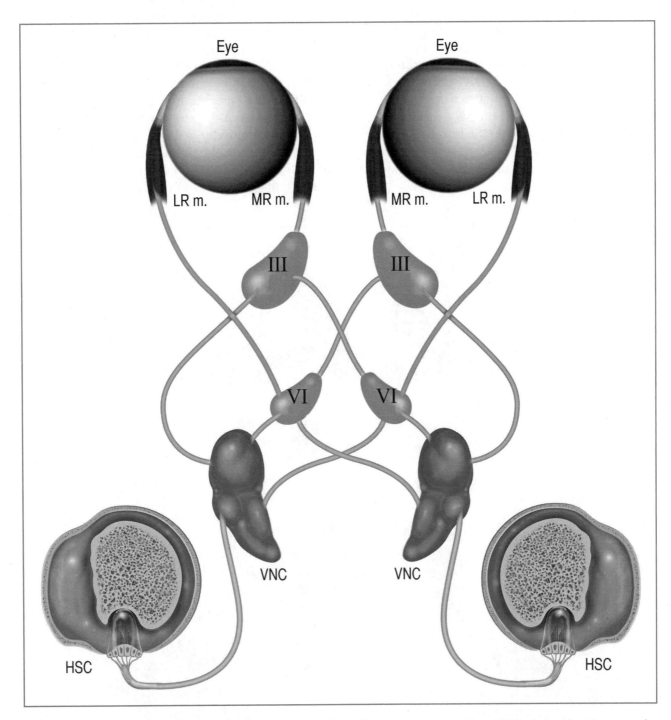

FIGURE 2–19. Direct pathway of the horizontal semicircular canal–ocular reflex. **LR m.** Lateral rectus muscle; **MR m.** medial rectus muscle; **HSC** horizontal semicircular canal; **VNC** vestibular nuclei complex; **III** oculomotor nucleus; **VI** abducens nucleus.

In our example of a head turn to the right, the left abducens nucleus and right oculomotor nucleus route the increased neural input received from the medial VN to the motor neurons of the left lateral rectus muscles and right medial rectus extraocular muscles. This pattern of input received by the EOMs initiates a contraction (i.e., shortening) of these two muscles resulting in the eye being pulled slowly to the left. This conjugate movement of the eyes to the left should be proportional to the size or magnitude of the head turn (Figure 2–20).

There is also a corresponding decrease in neural drive to the antagonist extraocular muscles (i.e., right lateral rectus and left medial rectus). The decrease in neural activity received by the left medial VN from the peripheral system is relayed to the left oculomotor nuclei and right abducens resulting in a relaxation of the left medial rectus and right lateral rectus muscles (Figure 2–21). These coordinated eye movements would not be possible without the medial longitudinal fasciculus (MLF). The MLF is the brainstem pathway that coordinates the outputs of the VN to the oculomo-

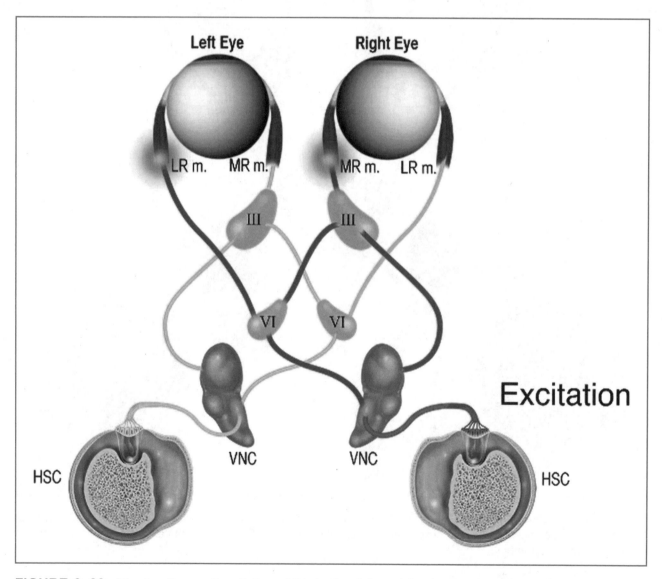

FIGURE 2–20. Direct pathway of excitation of the horizontal semicircular canal–ocular reflex during rotation of the head to the right. **LR m.** Lateral rectus muscle; **MR m.** medial rectus muscle; **HSC** horizontal semicircular canal; **VNC** vestibular nuclei complex; **III** oculomotor nucleus; **VI** abducens nucleus.

tor and abducens nuclei. This pathway makes it possible for these compensatory eye movements to be conjugate (i.e., for the visual axes to be parallel) (Figure 2–22).

In instances when an individual is subjected to a continuous rotation, the eyes are driven by the vestibular system to their lateral extremes in the orbits. When the eyes reach this critical point in the orbits, they must be reset to their original position and begin the deviation again or stop moving. If the eyes stop moving during the head movement, then the environment blurs due to the poor resolving capabilities of the retina. At this point, the eyes are able to be reset by specialized neurons in a distributed group of cells called the paramedian pontine reticular formation (PPRF). The PPRF briefly interrupts the flow of electrical activity from the vestibular periphery which allows the oculomotor system to initiate a saccade to send the eyes back to midline. The PPRF cells then go through a refractory cycle where input from the vestibular system is permitted once again

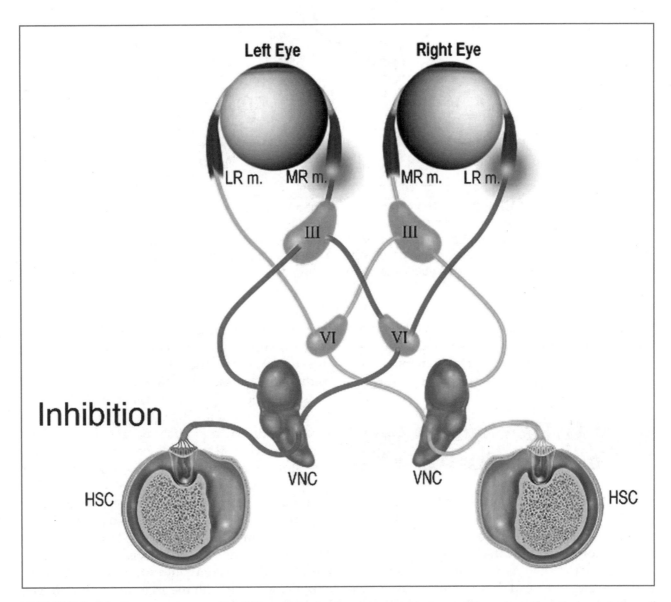

FIGURE 2–21. Direct pathway of inhibition of the horizontal semicircular canal–ocular reflex during rotation of the head to the right. **LR m.** Lateral rectus muscle; **MR m.** medial rectus muscle; **HSC** horizontal semicircular canal; **VNC** vestibular nuclei complex; **III** oculomotor nucleus; **VI** abducens nucleus.

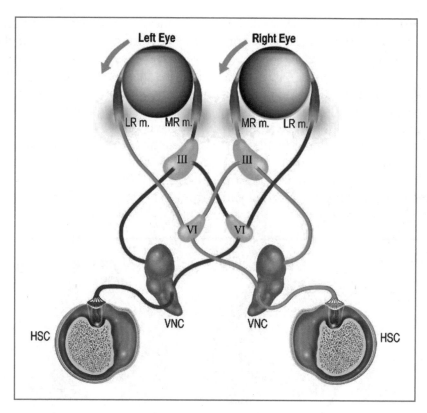

FIGURE 2–22. The complete series of events that occur in the horizontal semicircular canal–ocular reflex during rotation of the head to the right. **LR m.** Lateral rectus muscle; **MR m.** medial rectus muscle; **HSC** horizontal semicircular canal; **VNC** vestibular nuclei complex; **III** oculomotor nucleus; **VI** abducens nucleus.

to drive the eyes laterally. Again, this drive from the vestibular periphery is interrupted by neurons in the PPRF, and continues in this manner. This repetitive eye movement is called nystagmus.

VESTIBULAR NYSTAGMUS

While there are many forms of nystagmus, the one that is associated with the VOR is a normal response by the vestibular system to head acceleration. The reaction consists of producing a compensatory eye movement that is equal to, and opposite, the head movement followed by a quick movement of the eye in the opposite direction. Vestibular nystagmus generated by stimulation of the SCCs through angular acceleration

consists of two primary components. The first component is a slow deviation of the eyes in the direction opposite the head turn. This is known as the "slow phase." The slow phase is generated by the vestibular system and is the response of the VOR to acceleration. This is the component that is measured during quantitative assessment (caloric and rotary chair testing) of the horizontal canals. The slow phase is followed by a second faster component called the "fast phase" (Figure 2–23). Without a corrective movement of the eye in the opposite direction, the eye would reach the limits of the orbit and the VOR would stop functioning. The fast component of the VOR is not generated by the vestibular system, but rather by a pulse generator associated with the saccade system (PPRF). The PPRF is a distributed group of cells that are located near the abducens nuclei and have been shown to be active immediately prior to a fast phase being generated (Curthoys, 2002). It has been suggested that the PPRF monitors the ongoing VOR, and when the eye reaches a certain position in the orbit, burst neurons fire and quickly move the eye in the opposite direction. For angular accelerations, fast-phase nystagmus components have been shown to be larger than the slow-phase components. This would effectively put the eye in a position to acquire targets that are arriving (Baloh & Honrubia, 1990). An extensive review of the generation of the quick phase of vestibular nystagmus is presented in an article by Curthoys (2002).

It is possible for patients to have selective impairments in the PPRF that disrupt the ability to generate fast phases. Figure 2–24 compares the saccades of a neurologically intact patient with a patient who has a defect in the PPRF system. The impaired patient is incapable of producing the ballistic eye movements required for the generation of saccades. The patient was identified as having a saccade defect during the ENG/VNG test and was subsequently diagnosed by a neurologist as having a global saccadic palsy secondary to "progressive supranuclear palsy."

How Nystagmus Is Quantified

While it may seem counterintuitive, by convention, nystagmus is described by the direction of its fast phase. For instance, nystagmus with a fast phase to the right and a slow phase to the left would be said to be "right-beating." When the VOR is invoked during a movement of the head, the nystagmus typically beats in the direction of the head turn. There are several variables that can be used to quantify nystagmus; these include velocity, amplitude, latency, and duration (Jacobson, Newman, & Peterson,1993). In order to accurately measure nystagmus, the clinician must have an understanding of how the eye movements are being plotted during the recording. Specifically, the majority of commercial eye movement recorders plot eye movement (y axis) as a function of time (x axis). Most computerized systems allow the examiner to adjust the time scale while the calibration procedure determines the scale for the

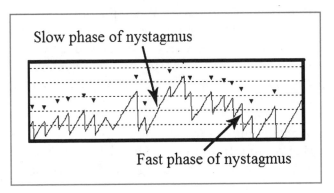

FIGURE 2–23. Nystagmus as recorded and displayed by an Interacoustics VNG system (Interacoustics, Assens, Denmark).

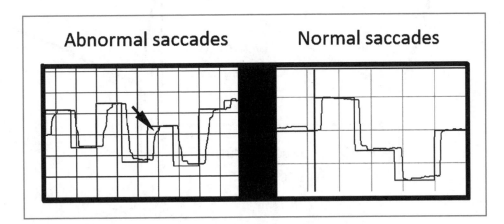

FIGURE 2–24. Saccades in a patient with a diagnosed "saccade defect" compared with saccades in a neurologically intact patient.

eye movement. The slow-phase velocity (SPV) of nystagmus is the most commonly used variable to quantify nystagmus and represents the amplitude of the response over a period of time (Figure 2–25). The SPV of nystagmus represents the distance that the eye moves during the slow phase divided by how long the eyes took to make the excursion. To measure the slow phase of a beat of nystagmus, most computerized systems incorporate a line that can be aligned with the slow phase and provide a measure of the slope. By convention, most systems use a time base of 1 s. The latency of the nystagmus, whether provoked by the caloric irrigation or another subtest during the examination, is the time it takes the response to occur once a test has been initiated. A measure of the frequency of the nystagmus can be obtained by counting the number of beats that occur during a specific time period.

THE VOR DURING SUSTAINED MOVEMENT

The VOR works to maintain clear vision during head movements and each head movement has a frequency; however, the vestibular system is not equally sensitive to all frequencies due to endolymph-cupular dynamics. The SCCs are less sensitive to angular accelerations below 0.05 Hz and above 3 Hz (Baloh & Honrubia, 2001). Furthermore, because the cupula is insensitive to gravity (the cupula and the endolymph have the same specific gravity), the vestibular system is poor at transducing sustained constant-velocity movements. Specifically, during a constant-velocity rotation, fluid motion approximates the speed of the canals and the cupula drifts back to its neutral position, and peripheral drive to the central nervous system ceases (Goldberg & Fernandez, 1971a). In order to compensate for the fact that the VOR is poor at transducing low-frequency accelerations and sustained constant-velocity rotations, the vestibular system has a central nervous system function that enhances its sensitivity during these dynamic situations. When the time constant (time taken for a response to decay to 37% of its initial value) of the VOR is measured in response to a sustained rotational stimulus, the nystagmus persists approximately three times longer than the "drive" from the periphery (Raphan, Matsuo, & Cohen, 1979). This extension of the VOR response past the point where there is no longer any neural drive coming from the peripheral end organs has been termed "velocity storage" (VS). VS is medi-

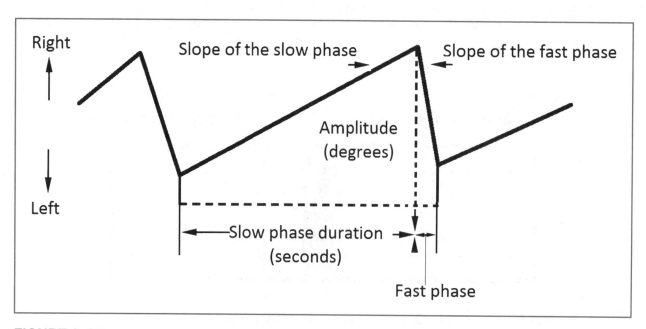

FIGURE 2–25. The variables of nystagmus that can be measured. (Redrawn from Jacobson, Newman, and Kartush, 1993)

ated by a distributed system of neural structures which are collectively termed the "neural integrator" (NI) (Leigh & Zee, 2006). These structures include the VN, commissural fibers connecting the VN, and the connections between VN and the cerebellum.

The NI facilitates the process of VS in two primary ways. First, the NI collects and stores electrical activity arriving from the primary vestibular afferents. In this way it acts as a capacitor (i.e., a circuit that stores a charge). Second, the NI gates the outflow of electrical activity that it has collected. The amount of neural activity that the NI releases from its "storage bank" is dependent on the type of movement being encountered and whether or not the peripheral vestibular system is impaired. The primary purpose of VS is to extend the time constant of the VOR one order of magnitude beyond what the canal responses produce during low-frequency or constant-velocity rotations. The centrally mediated prolongation of the nystagmus after the canal responses have ceased providing input effectively extends the low-frequency response of the vestibular system; however, it has been reported that in cases of peripheral vestibular system impairment, the VS mechanism opens the valve and significantly increases the outflow. The VS mechanism is implicated in several tests used to assess the vestibular system (e.g., headshake and rotational testing). In fact, it has been reported that patients with impairments in the VS mechanism may contribute to balance impairments in unsteady, fall-prone patients. (Jacobson & McCaslin, 2004).

3

Peripheral Vestibular Impairment and Central Nervous System Compensation

INTRODUCTION

When a person with two healthy peripheral vestibular systems suddenly loses function in one of them, they manifest a distinct pattern of symptoms. First, the patient complains of "true" vertigo defined as the entire environment rotating around the patient or the patient turning inside the environment. They may also describe experiencing nausea and vomiting. Second, if the patient's vestibular impairment is acute, they manifest a primarily linear horizontal nystagmus with the quick phase directed away from the impaired ear. This nystagmus typically enhances when the patient is unable to fixate (e.g., when the nystagmus is observed using video goggles and vision is denied.) Third, the patient demonstrates postural impairments, such as falling to the affected side, or they may complain that they experience difficulty walking straight or are very unstable in environments that are poorly lit. Interestingly, in neurologically intact individuals these symptoms begin to subside within a week. After the vertigo has stopped, patients may still complain of feeling

strange when making quick head movements, but typically within less than a month they are able to resume their pre-attack lifestyle. This ability for the vestibular system to recover following an insult to the peripheral end organ or vestibular nerves has been termed "vestibular compensation" or "vestibular adaptation." It is vital for the clinicians administering VNG examinations to understand the neural basis of the phenomenon and its effect on the various subtests of the VNG.

EFFECT OF UNILATERAL VESTIBULAR LESIONS

In order to understand what happens in the case of a peripheral vestibular system impairment, one must have an understanding of what happens in an intact system. Figure 3–1 shows that when a person turns their head to the left, there is an increase in tonic neural activity on the left side (i.e., in the direction of the head turn) and a corresponding decrease in activity on the right side (i.e., the side contralateral to the head turn). As is explained in Chapter 2 (see the description

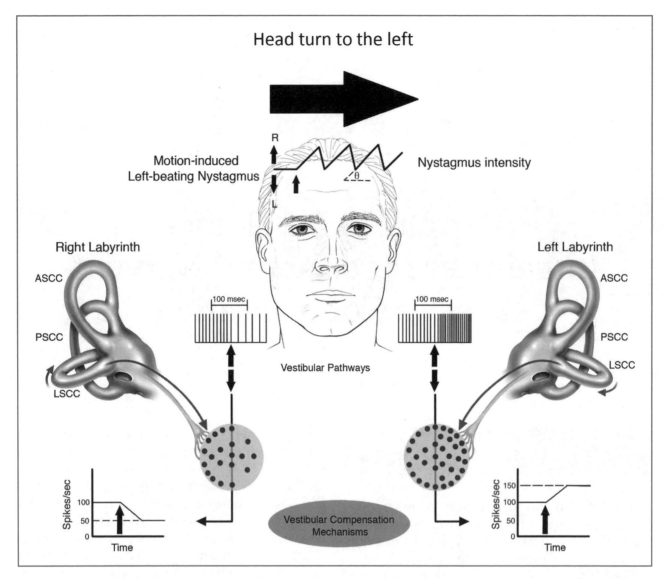

FIGURE 3–1. The change in primary afferent firing rate and resulting eye movement following rotation of the head to the left. The *circle* represents the vestibular nuclei and the number of *dots* the level of neural activity. **ASCC** anterior semicircular canal; **PSCC** posterior semicircular canal; **LSCC** lateral semicircular canal. (Adapted from Barin & Durrant, 2000)

of the vestibuloocular reflex [VOR]), this type of head turn produces an asymmetry in the neural drive from the peripheral vestibular system. This peripherally generated asymmetrical neural drive is relayed through the oculomotor neurons to the extraocular muscles. The pattern of neural activity received by the motor system produces the aforementioned slow eye movement in the opposite direction of the head turn that is proportional to the velocity of the head movement. Once the eye reaches a specific point in the orbit, the vestibular

input is blocked briefly allowing the oculomotor system to reset the eye in the direction of the head movement (i.e., nystagmus).

Damage to one of the peripheral vestibular end organs or vestibular nerves can occur for several reasons. For example, there may be a disease process that injures the hair cells in the labyrinth or destroys neurons in the nerve. An illustration of what happens physiologically when a person incurs a loss of function of one of their peripheral vestibular systems is presented in Figure 3–2. As

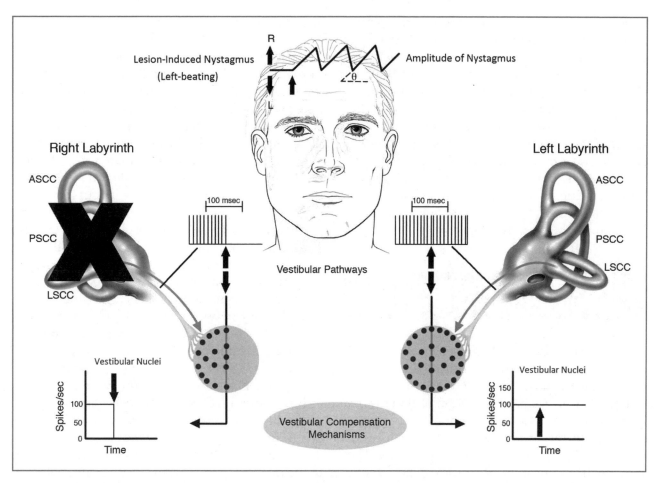

FIGURE 3–2. The change in primary afferent firing rate and resulting eye movement following an acute loss of peripheral vestibular function on the right side. **ASCC** anterior semicircular canal; **PSCC** posterior semicircular canal; **LSCC** lateral semicircular canal. (Adapted from Barin & Durrant, 2000)

can be seen from the figure, there is a significant decrease in the tonic activity from the right peripheral system routed to the vestibular nuclei. This asymmetry in tonic neural activity generates an electrical "code" that the brain falsely interprets as a head turn. In fact, during the acute phase following a loss of peripheral vestibular function, the patient perceives that they are turning toward the healthy ear. It is this false perception of rotation generated by the loss of peripheral vestibular function that has been termed vertigo. In addition to the perception of rotary motion, patients may also experience vegetative symptoms. The tonic neural asymmetry results in a sensory "mismatch" between information that the vestibular system is providing (i.e., patient is turning) compared with other supporting senses (e.g., somesthetic system

and vision) that the patient is, in fact, sitting still. The patient experiences autonomic system symptoms of pallor, sweating, nausea, and vomiting.

The perception of vertigo is a product of the aberrant nystagmus (i.e., spontaneous vestibular nystagmus) generated by the asymmetry registered at the vestibular nuclei. In a normally functioning vestibular system, when the head is moved the VOR drives the eyes in an equal and opposite direction. This stabilizes the environment and the perception of movement is mitigated; however, in the case of a loss of vestibular function on one side, the head is static, but nystagmus is generated due to the tonic neural asymmetry. Because the eyes are moving (i.e., spontaneous nystagmus) in the absence of any head movement, the perception of the patient is that of rotation. The nystagmus generated by the loss of function in the peripheral vestibular system is primarily (although not entirely) horizontally linear and is a direct result of the loss of neural tonic input from the impaired side. The reason that the nystagmus is not purely horizontal is that the input from the two vertical canals (i.e., posterior and anterior) cancels out incompletely leaving a small residual torsional component. Acutely, the slow component of the nystagmus is directed toward the impaired ear; however, due to compensation mechanisms, the direction of the nystagmus is not always a reliable indicator of the impaired ear.

NEURAL BASIS OF VESTIBULAR COMPENSATION

The vestibular system has an elegant adaptive mechanism that is activated during an acute loss of vestibular input from one side. In situations where there is an extended asymmetry in the neural firing rate due to impairment of the peripheral system, central vestibular system structures are first recruited to eliminate the asymmetry. Then they begin the process of restoring the dynamic function of the VOR. This process is termed "vestibular compensation" and consists of two primary stages. The first stage consists of eliminating symptoms such as spontaneous nystagmus and skew deviation by rebalancing the tonic neural activity in the vestibular nuclei. This stage has been referred to in the literature as "static compensation." The second stage is much more subtle, takes longer, and has been termed "dynamic compensation." Dynamic compensation involves a central recalibration of the response properties of the VOR (i.e., timing and gain) in order to restore the compensatory actions of the VOR to preimpairment levels. A patient's stage of compensation can have dramatic effects on the results of the various VNG subtests, and thus an understanding of the underlying mechanisms of compensation is important for all clinicians.

The following two sections outline the processes that occur during static and dynamic compensation in a simplified manner.

Static Compensation

The process of static compensation occurs almost immediately following unilateral vestibular deafferentation (uVD). This process consists of compensation mechanisms restoring the static balance in tonic neural activity between the vestibular systems. In other words, the asymmetry between the vestibular end organs is eliminated and there is no spontaneous vestibular nystagmus when the patient is not moving. As was discussed previously, each vestibular nerve routes a large amount of neural activity into the vestibular nuclei (VN) (e.g., 1,000,000 spikes per second). Following uVD, one of the VN ceases to receive this input resulting in an asymmetrical tonic neural resting rate between the two sides. The difference in neural input between the two VNs triggers the VOR into action thereby producing an aberrant nystagmus known as "spontaneous vestibular nystagmus" (SVN). Acutely, the fast phase of the nystagmus beats away the impaired ear. As soon as hours after uVD occurs, a phenomenon known in the literature as "cerebellar clamping" is initiated (Figure 3–3).

Midline cerebellar structures quickly respond to the imbalance in the tonic resting rates between the two VNs and increase the tonic inhibition in the contralesional VN. This increase in inhibition acts to decrease the tonic resting rate of the VN on the intact side, and as a consequence of this, the asymmetry between the two VNs is reduced (or clamped). The process not only reduces the amplitude of the SVN (decrease in the severity of the vertigo), but also the severity of the symptoms generated by the autonomic nervous system such as nausea and pallor. At this point the neural tonic resting rate of both VN is reduced compared with levels before the insult. In fact, if a patient is tested using caloric or rotational stimuli, they often manifest findings consistent with a bilateral peripheral vestibular impairment. The process of cerebellar clamping is more complex than presented here, and a more detailed account of the process is given by Curthoys and Halmagyi (1996). Once the activity to the contralesional VN has been "clamped," the next stage in the process of static compensation begins. In order to regain normal perfor-

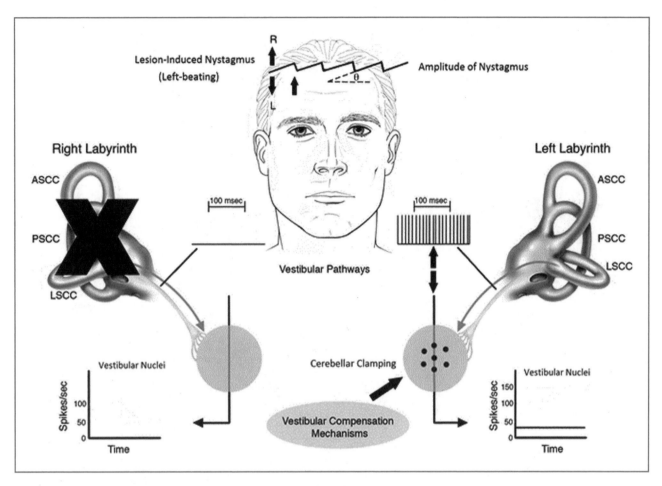

FIGURE 3–3. An illustration of how "cerebellar clamping" of the vestibular nuclei reduces the intensity of spontaneous vestibular nystagmus. **ASCC** anterior semicircular canal; **PSCC** posterior semicircular canal; **LSCC** lateral semicircular canal. (Adapted from Barin & Durrant, 2000)

mance of the VOR, the neural resting rates of both VN need to be brought back to their original levels. First, the level of clamping must be reduced on the intact side. In order to accomplish that task, the midline cerebellum decreases the level of neural drive sent through its direct inhibitory connections to the VN. This effectively increases the level of neural tonic firing rate (i.e., reduces inhibition) in the contralesional VN and releases it from its "clamped" state (Figure 3–4).

Second, the tonic resting rate must be restored on the impaired side. Reports have shown that as soon as 52 hours following uVD, the neural resting rate in the ipsilesional VN can be equivalent to rates that preceded the insult (Curthoys & Halmagyi, 1996). This increase in the tonic firing rate

in the ipsilesional VN has been suggested to have several different origins with the primary one being a release of inhibition mediated by the midline cerebellum (Jacobson, Pearlstein, Henderson, Calder, & Rock, 1998). The process of static compensation is completed when the neural resting rates in the two VN are equilibrated (Figure 3–5).

Dynamic Compensation

Following the process of static compensation, the dynamic response properties of the VOR remain impaired. Specifically, compensation mechanisms modify the properties of the central vestibular system to account for the fact that the impaired

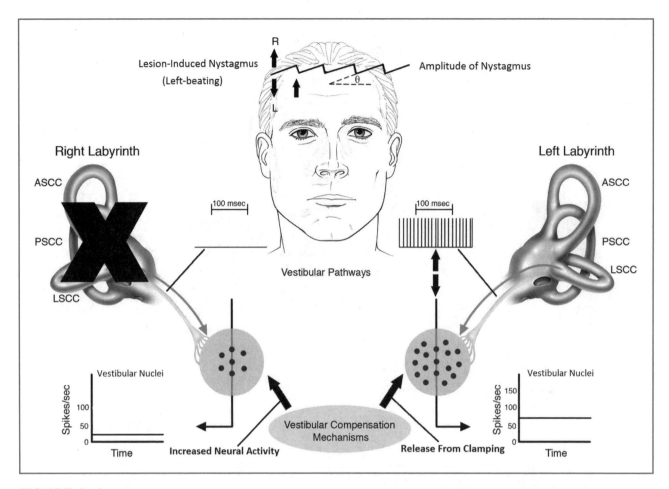

FIGURE 3–4. An illustration of how the cerebellum releases the "clamping" on the intact side and increases neural activity at the level of the vestibular nuclei on the impaired side. **ASCC** anterior semicircular canal; **PSCC** posterior semicircular canal; **LSCC** lateral semicircular canal. (Adapted from Barin & Durrant, 2000)

organ does not produce the appropriate neural drive during head movements. The tonic resting rate of the two VNs is equal at this stage; however, in the case of head movements there is little or no increase in neural input from the ipsilesional peripheral system. The VOR response is at this point only receiving drive from one labyrinth and cannot provide accurate compensatory eye movements during dynamic situations. The process of dynamic compensation consists of central structures adjusting the vestibular systems neural output to accurately drive the VOR with only one labyrinth (Figure 3–6).

Two of the primary facilitators of dynamic compensation are visual input (Leigh & Zee, 2006) and the midline cerebellum (Beraneck, McKee, Aleisa, & Cullen, 2008). While research has shown that together these two systems play a critical role in the recovery of VOR function after uVD, there are other contributors (e.g., commissural fibers between the VN and spinal input). The ability of this process to completely restore dynamic function is also dependent on the severity of the impairment. In complete or severe uVDs there are often permanent decrements in VOR performance. In such cases , the compensation process makes sacrifices in the response characteristics of the VOR in order to maximize performance in frequencies critical for functioning. For example, the neural integrator decreases the amount of neural activity held by the velocity storage mechanism (low frequency) and allocates it to frequencies

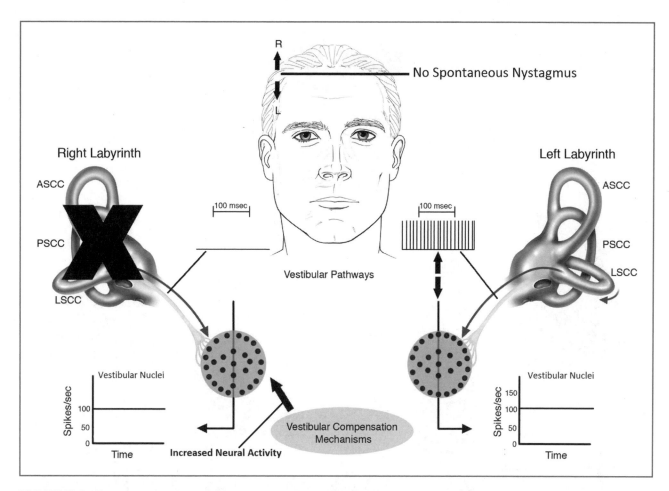

FIGURE 3–5. The level of activity at the peripheral vestibular afferents and vestibular nuclei following static compensation. Note that there is no longer any spontaneous vestibular nystagmus. **ASCC** anterior semicircular canal; **PSCC** posterior semicircular canal; **LSCC** lateral semicircular canal. (Adapted from Barin & Durrant, 2000)

encountered during ambulation (high frequency). These adjustments to the central vestibular system that occur during dynamic compensation following uVD often result in permanent abnormalities in the VOR at high accelerations and sensitivity to low-frequency stimuli (Leigh & Zee, 2006; Barin & Durrant, 2000).

Recovery Nystagmus

Occasionally, in patients with irritative (fluctuating) vestibular impairments (e.g., Ménière disease), a phenomenon known as recovery nystagmus (RN) is observed. This form of spontaneous nystagmus has also been referred to as

"Bechterew's" nystagmus and is characterized by the fast-phase beating toward the ipsilesional ear (Leigh & Zee, 2006; Jacobson et al., 1998). Clinically, RN can be difficult to interpret because in cases where the impaired ear is clearly identified, the nystagmus appears to be beating in a paradoxical direction (fast phase toward the impaired ear). When a lesion affecting one inner ear of balance is stable, compensation mechanisms are highly effective; however, in cases where the function of the impaired vestibular system fluctuates, central compensation mechanisms need to adjust accordingly. An example of this would be when a patient has active Ménière disease. Acutely, following an attack, the patient demonstrates a spontaneous nystagmus where the fast phase beats toward the

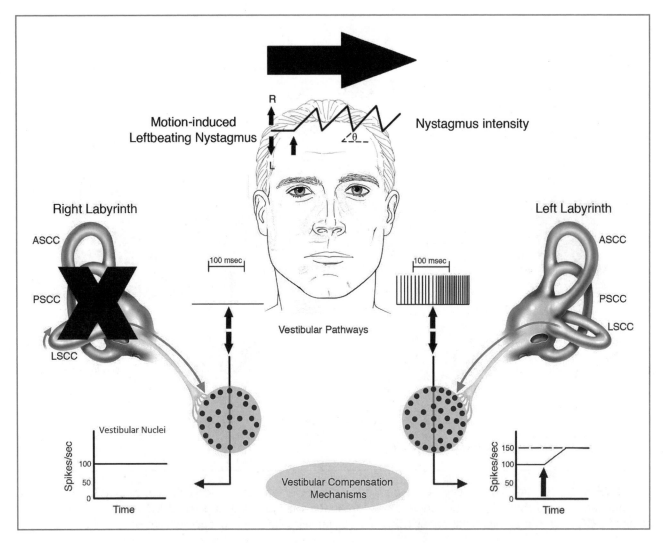

FIGURE 3–6. The change in primary afferent firing rate and resulting eye movement following rotation of the head to the left after the patient has achieved dynamic compensation. **ASCC** anterior semicircular canal; **PSCC** posterior semicircular canal; **LSCC** lateral semicircular canal. (Adapted from Barin & Durrant, 2000)

intact ear. The presence of the persistent neural asymmetry between the two end organs triggers central nervous system compensation mechanisms to become active and the asymmetry is reduced by cerebellar clamping (Figure 3–7). RN is most commonly observed during the "clamping" phase of compensation or when the level of neural activity at the VN is reduced bilaterally. At this stage in the compensation process, if there is a recovery of function on the impaired side, it will create another tonic neural asymmetry, only this time in the opposite direction. Given that the level of tonic activity in the vestibular nucleus on the intact side has been reduced, a recovery of function in the previously impaired ear raises the tonic neural output of the impaired ear over that of the healthy ear. This set of circumstances generates a spontaneous nystagmus where the fast phase beats toward the impaired but recovering ear. If the recovery of the ear is stable, the patient should statically compensate and the RN will disappear. It is critical that the clinician understand the circumstances and characteristics of RN so as to avoid any misinterpretation during ENG/VNG examination. Because of the unstable nature of some disease processes and the dynamic nature of central

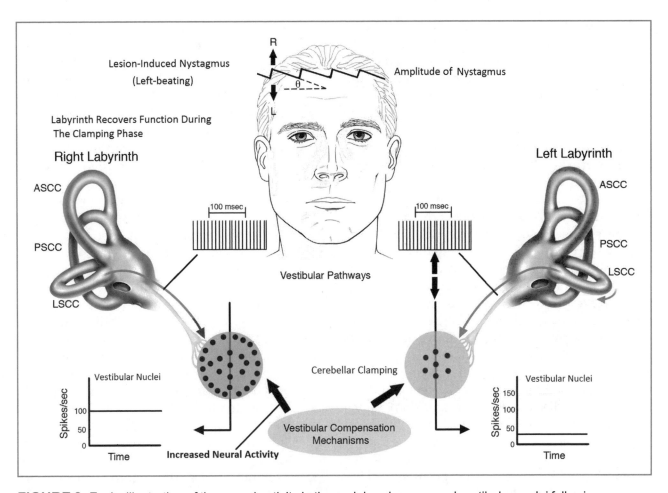

FIGURE 3–7. An illustration of the neural activity in the peripheral nerves and vestibular nuclei following recovery of function to the impaired labyrinth. Note that the nystagmus beats in the opposite direction from the previous examples (i.e., recovery nystagmus). **ASCC** anterior semicircular canal; **PSCC** posterior semicircular canal; **LSCC** lateral semicircular canal. (Adapted from Barin & Durrant, 2000)

nervous system compensation, the clinician cannot always rely on the direction of the nystagmus to identify the impaired ear. A comprehensive review of RN is given by Jacobson et al. (1998).

LAWS OF COMPENSATION

Vestibular compensation is most effective when the following conditions are met:

1. Patients are not taking vestibular suppressants.
2. Patients must move their heads (a basic tenant of vestibular rehabilitation therapy).

3. Patients have intact vestibular pathways.
4. Patients have vision.

CALORIC STIMULATION OF THE VESTIBULAR SYSTEM

As is described in Chapter 1, the vestibular system is naturally sensitive to head movements; however, many quantitative vestibular assessments utilize nonphysiologic stimuli (e.g., acoustic or thermal) to evoke calibrated responses from the end organs. With regard to the caloric test, it was Robert Barany in 1907 who first provided a description of how to do the caloric test and the hypothesis that described the underlying mechanism of how it stimulated the inner ear of balance (Hood, 1989). When water with a temperature above or below normal body temperature is infused into the external auditory meatus, the temperature of the skin and tympanic membrane is either warmed or cooled. The lateral semicircular canal is sensitive to any temperature variations in the external auditory canal because of its close proximity to the middle ear space. Specifically, any change in temperature from normal body temperature is conducted through the middle ear space to the vestibule (Harrington, 1969). The physiologic mechanism underlying this test is that the temperature gradient induced by the irrigation results in a change in the specific gravity of the endolymph in the lateral semicircular canal on the side that is irrigated. The clever ability to unilaterally drive the firing rate above or below its baseline using a medium of different temperatures enables the clinician to generate asymmetries in the firing rates of the vestibular system and drive the VOR, as is discussed in Chapter 2. In Barany's original description of the caloric test, he noted that the test should be performed with the patient supine and the head elevated 30° (Figure 3–8A). When the head is oriented in this position, or if the head is flexed 60° backward, the lateral semicircular canals are oriented vertically and placed in line with the gravity vector.

When the medium that has a temperature higher or lower than the body is introduced into the external auditory canal, the endolymph in the part of the lateral canal closest to the middle ear space is heated. When a fluid is heated its density is lowered. A good example of this is when water is boiled. As the water is heated and begins to boil, it turns into steam and rises. So heat lowers the density of the water (makes it less heavy) and causes it to rise (Figure 3–8B). In the case of the caloric examination, the heat is diffused through the middle ear space and heats the endolymph in the portion of the lateral canal closest to the irrigation. As the heated endolymph rises, it is replaced by cooler (more dense) endolymph which is in turn heated and its density lowered. This process of fluid motion, termed "convection current," goes on until the irrigation (stimulus) is terminated.

Introduction of a warm medium results in an excitatory response in the labyrinth on the side of the irrigation. As is described in Chapter 2, the cupula in the lateral semicircular canal has the same density as the surrounding endolymph, and the stereocilia that are embedded into the base of it are all oriented toward the utricle. Figure 3–9A illustrates what happens when we infuse a warm-water stimulus into the external ear on the left side. As the endolymph near the middle ear space becomes lighter it rises. This in turn pushes cupula toward the utricle, depolarizing the hair cells in the cristae, and increases the tonic resting rate in the nerve above its baseline activity. This direction of movement of the cupula in the lateral semicircular canal has been termed "utriculopetal" and it

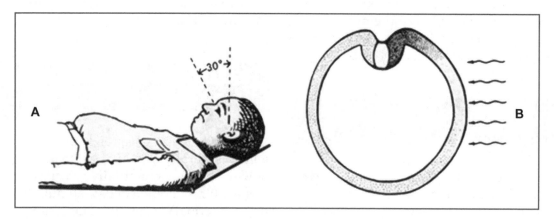

FIGURE 3–8. A. The 30° supine position for caloric testing that places the horizontal canals into a vertical position for maximal stimulation during caloric testing. B. An illustration of how endolymph rises during a warm caloric irrigation. (From Barber & Stockwell, 1976)

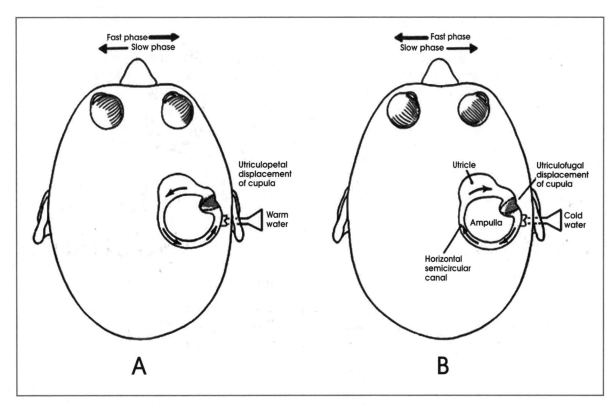

FIGURE 3–9. The movement of endolymph in the lateral semicircular canal and the associated eye movements following a cool and warm caloric irrigation. (From Baloh, 1998b)

mimics a head turn toward the irrigated ear (excitatory). With this type of response a nystagmus is generated with fast phases beating toward the ear being irrigated.

In the case of a cool irrigation, the density of the endolymph is increased (becomes heavier) and it begins to sink where it is, and then it is replaced by lighter endolymph again setting up a convection current, only this time in the opposite direction (Figure 3–9B). This type of endolymph movement deflects the cupula away from the utricle which initiates a hyperpolarization (inhibitory) of the cells in the cristae on the irrigated side and a corresponding decrease in the firing rate of the vestibular nerve below its baseline resting rate. The deflection of the cupula away from the utricle has been termed "uticulofugal" and mimics a head turn away from the stimulated side. The VOR response in this case is a nystagmus with the fast phase beating away from the irrigated ear. One easy way to remember the relationship between the temperature and the direction of the

nystagmus is to employ the mnemonic "COWS": Cold–Opposite–Warm–Same.

For the most part, Barany's original hypothesis set forth in 1907 is correct; however, experiments following his initial explanations of the caloric effect have modified to some degree the theory regarding the exact mechanism. There is no question that the change in the density of the endolymph is a major contributor to the generation of the response. In an elegant series of experiments, Coats and Smith (1967) showed that the caloric response reverses when a patient is tested with their face pointing toward the ground (prone) versus lying on their back (supine). In the prone position, the lateral canals are also oriented vertically, only this time they are inverted with respect to the supine position described previously. If a medium of sufficient temperature is introduced into the external auditory meatus, the portion of the lateral canal nearest the middle ear space is heated. As in the supine position, the endolymph becomes lighter, starts to rise, and presses on the cupula. When the subject is in the prone position, an upward movement of the cupula bends it away from the utricle and the characteristics of the vestibular nystagmus are such that the fast phase beats away from the irrigated ear. Furthermore, when a cool irrigation is administered with the patient in the prone position, a nystagmus with the fast phase beating toward the irrigated ear can be observed. Coats and Smith (1967) reported this reversal of the caloric response in different head positions further confirming Barany's original

hypothesis that the caloric response is dependent on gravity. The frequency of the caloric stimulus has been calculated to be approximately 0.003 Hz. Figure 3–10 shows a slow-phase velocity profile of a caloric response and illustrates the support for this assertion. The time course for the caloric-induced nystagmus, beginning with the onset of the nystagmus to where it disappears, is approximately 140 s. The velocity profile of one caloric response could represent a half cycle of a sine wave, and thus a full cycle would be twice as

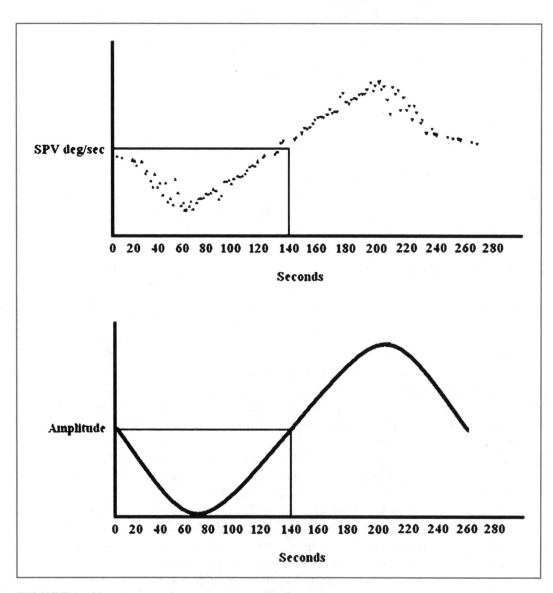

FIGURE 3–10. Illustration of a velocity profile of a caloric response showing the origin of the assertion that a caloric stimulus results in a response akin to a rotational frequency of 0.003 Hz. SPV, slow-phase velocity. (From McCaslin and Jacobson, 2009)

much (280 s). The reciprocal of 280 s is 0.004 Hz, which is very close to the reported 0.003 Hz.

Coats and Smith (1967) also reported a difference in the amplitude of the response with head position. Specifically, the authors suggested that there is a second contributor to the caloric response that is not dependent on gravity. The authors proposed that this secondary component of transduction within the lateral canal system is associated with thermal stimulation of the vestibular nerve itself. To further explore this concept, the origin of caloric stimulation warranted its own experiment on the Spacelab-I, which was a laboratory that traveled in the space shuttle's cargo bay. This allowed the caloric response to be evaluated in a weightless atmosphere. The idea was that if changing the weight of the endolymph is the only source of the caloric response, then in a zero-gravity environment there should be an absent response. In fact, caloric nystagmus was elicited in space following an irrigation proving that there are additional contributors to the response (e.g., firing rate of the nerve is increased when it is exposed to a temperature warmer or cooler than body temperature) (Scherer, Brandt, Clarke, Merbold, & Parker, 1986).

||| 4 |||

Pretest Procedures for VNG

INTRODUCTION

When the clinician first greets the patient in the waiting room, the examination has officially begun. The examiner should introduce himself or herself and always ask the patient if there is someone that they would like to accompany them during the testing. This is an important question because many patients with vertigo have a misunderstanding or distorted perception of what is going to happen during the VNG test. Having a family member or friend with them during the examination can greatly reduce the patient's level of anxiety and increase the quality of the data collected. At this stage of the interview, the examiner should note if the patient is in a wheelchair, hearing impaired, or visually impaired. In cases where a patient is severely hearing impaired, he or she should be made aware that it is okay to wear hearing aids or activate their cochlear implant. If a patient is severely visually impaired, the clinician needs to determine if calibration is possible. If the patient is blind, caloric testing can still be completed using a default calibration; however, only statements about whether or not the patient has vestibular function can be made. Given that the system will essentially be uncalibrated for the patient, conventional quantitative measures derived from the caloric testing cannot be employed (e.g., unilateral weakness and directional preponderance). The clinician should also be vigilant to the presence of "blind nystagmus" in patients with severe visual impairments. Prior to doing any testing, a thorough case history, otoscopic examination, and gross eye movement evaluation should be conducted.

CASE HISTORY

Agarwal and colleagues (2009) estimate that 24–60 million people experience symptoms of vestibular impairment during their lifetime. It has been estimated that dizziness is the presenting complaint in 2.5% of patients who are evaluated by primary care physicians each year (Sloane, 1989). If this is true, then primary care physicians evaluate over 8 million dizzy/vertiginous/unsteady patients per year. It is estimated that 26% of the 8 million dizzy patients are unable to work because of dizziness, and this results in a financial impact of $2.25 billion (assuming that the dizziness results in $30,000 per person in economic damage from medical claims, health insurance, and disability payments). Dizziness and vertigo also represented 2–3% of all emergency department consultations from 1995 to 2004 (Kerber et al., 2008). This amounted to 26 million visits to emergency departments in the United States for dizziness during that time span. Additionally, it probably is not surprising that when patients are evaluated in either the emergency department or the primary care setting, the final diagnoses are more often general medical diagnoses (e.g., hypertension, elevated blood glucose, and coronary artery disease) compared with the final diagnoses when the same patients are evaluated by ear specialists.

Case history taking in the assessment of the dizzy/unsteady patient can be a frustrating experience for both the clinician and the patient. The clinician must attempt to acquire from the patient salient pieces of information in a short period of time. The clinician must synthesize this information as it is being acquired so that the examination of the patient (e.g., the choice of examinations) can be tailored to the patient's complaints. The case history also enables the clinician to generate hypotheses about the source of the patient's complaints (i.e., the differential diagnosis), which are either supported or not supported by the results of objective tests (e.g., neuroimaging, electroneurodiagnostic tests). Often patients complicate the history-taking process by recounting what they feel is valuable information that, in fact, contributes little to the differential diagnosis. Patients may feel that they have been ignored if they are not given sufficient time to provide the clinician with information. Despite these shortcomings, many clinicians believe that a well-conducted case history is the most important part of dizziness assessment (e.g., Baloh & Honrubia, 2001).

Dizziness is similar to other medical problems in that a thorough case history (qualitative information) paired with laboratory testing (quantitative testing) can help confirm the underlying etiology of the impairment; thus, it is crucial that adequate time for the case history be allotted during the examination. Prior to the interview the examiner should have reviewed the patient's past medical history. This enables the examiner to determine if there are any predisposing factors that may be contributing to the condition of the patient. The formal case history is typically conducted at the beginning of the assessment, but it can also begin prior to the appointment. Patients

may be sent structured questionnaires to their home so that the forms can be filled out with the help of a significant other and with no time limitation. (An example of a dizziness case history form is included in Appendix A.) In this regard patients can begin to organize the occurrences and triggers of their dizziness which will facilitate the interview with the examiner; however, a face-to-face systematic interview is often most useful because it affords the patient to describe the symptoms in his or her own words. This can often help the interviewer categorize the nature of the complaints or sensations and direct the interview in a meaningful way. At the time of the appointment it should be determined if the patient would like any accompanying family members or friends to be present during the testing. This helps to put the patient at ease, and also occasionally the person accompanying the patient can provide additional information regarding the dizziness. When taking a case history the clinician should be seated directly across from the patient and ask questions that allow for interpretation. While there is a standard set of questions that are related to dizziness, the patient should be encouraged to provide a description of the symptoms in their own words. It is important that the questions help the clinician to better understand the nature of the patient's sensations as well as engage the patient in a historical account of when the dizziness started and what the status of it is at the time of the interview.

The following section presents questions that are often used to categorize information obtained from patients suffering from dizziness. Counseling materials created by the author and Gary P. Jacobson as well as a case history form developed by Joseph Furman and Stephen Cass can be found in Appendices A, B, and C.

Key Questions

The key questions to ask are given below.

Question 1: Can you describe the sensations that you are experiencing?

Question 2: How long does the dizziness last?

Question 3: Can you make the dizziness happen?

Question 4: Are there any other symptoms that accompany the dizziness?

Question 5: Do you have any other medical conditions?

Question 6: What medications are you taking?

Question 1: Can You Describe the Sensations that You Are Experiencing?

A good way to start the interview is to ask the patient to describe their symptoms. "Dizziness" is an imprecise term that patients often use to describe a number of different symptoms they are experiencing. For example, the symptoms the patient describes may be a feeling of floating or being lightheaded. The patient may also complain of vertigo, which is defined as "the sensation of motion when no motion is occurring relative to earth's gravity" (American Academy of Otolaryngology–HNS, 1995). The first step in a case history is to ask the patient to describe in their own words the sensations they are experiencing. It is common for the patient with dizziness to have more than one symptom. For instance, a patient may complain of a sensation of rotary motion accompanied by severe imbalance. The clinician should follow up with questions regarding what the impact of the sensations is on the patient's everyday activities and whether they change over time (e.g., "worse when I get up in the morning"). Occasionally patients have difficulty describing the symptoms and the examiner can direct the interview with questions such as "Are you unsteady?" or "Do the sensations feel like they are in your head?" During this initial part of the case history the clinician should be guiding the questioning and patient descriptions of what they are experiencing in a way that differentiates symptoms of vertigo from those of non-vertigo. According to Baloh and Honrubia (1990) less than 50% of patients who present with dizziness have true vertigo (Tables 4–1 and 4–2).

Question 2: How Long Does the Dizziness Last?

Following a description of the symptoms the examiner should begin determining the time course of the sensations. For example, is the patient experi-

Table 4–1. Symptoms and Sensations Related to Vertigo

Symptoms
The illusion of movement that usually is rotational (e.g., spinning) but can also be linear displacement (e.g., linear movement, tilt)
Sensations
"I feel like the room is spinning." (subjective vertigo)
"The room is spinning around me." (objective vertigo)
"I feel like I am shifting or falling." (subjective vertigo)

Table 4–2. Symptoms and Sensations Not Related to Vertigo

Symptoms
Panic attacks, persistent sensation of rocking in the absence of any movement, hyperventilation, motion sickness
Imbalance or unsteadiness while ambulating or standing
Lightheadedness or presyncope
Sensations
"When I sit and think about my problems I get dizzy."
"I have trouble focusing my eyes."
"I feel lightheaded."

encing dizziness that is episodic or is it constant? If it is episodic, then the clinician should ascertain how often the episodes occur (e.g., every day or once a month) and how long they last (e.g., seconds or hours). Is the patient free of symptoms between the spells? When conducting a case history with a patient experiencing episodic dizziness it is important to have them describe the characteristics of the initial symptom(s) (first attack) and their last attack. Understanding the characteristics of the first and last bouts of dizziness enable the clinician to make a determination as to whether spells are related or if they are independent of one another. In the latter case, a specific history may need to be taken and developed for each of the complaints. An example of this would be a patient who initially experienced a spontaneous attack of rotational vertigo and nausea that lasted for a day and then complained of dizziness only when lying down or sitting up in bed. In patients with persistent dizziness, the clinician should question the patient as to when the initial symptoms became evident and whether the dizziness seems to be getting progressively worse, resolving, or staying the same. Table 4–3 is an adaption from Bennett (2008) that pairs common disorders and their time course.

Question 3: Can You Make the Dizziness Happen?

Determining if there is anything a patient can do to provoke the symptoms or whether they are spontaneous is another key question in understanding the nature of the dizziness. The inquiry into what the circumstances are when the dizziness occurs should follow the description by the patient about the symptoms and their duration. For example, can the patient bring on the dizziness by performing a certain head movement? If a patient stands up and feels lightheaded, it may indicate a form of presyncope or positioning vertigo. Alternatively, a patient may have had an attack of vertigo that lasted anywhere from a day to a month and he or she continues to be very unstable during everyday activities. One method of helping to further discern the cause of dizziness is to pair the time course of the dizziness (question 2) with circumstances that provoke it (Bennett, 2008). This can help the examiner begin to classify the possible origin of the sensations that the patient is experiencing (Table 4–4).

Question 4: Are There Any Symptoms that Accompany the Dizziness?

Due to the proximity of the hearing and balance organs to one another, it is important that the clinician inquire about any otological symptoms that are concomitant with the dizziness. Patients who have disorders affecting the inner ear may present with tinnitus, hearing loss, and pain or pressure. Alternatively, patients may also have associated symptoms that are neurological. Impairments in the brain or central nervous system commonly manifest symptoms of dizziness. Disorders such as neoplasms, multiple sclerosis, cerebellar degenerations, and migraine can all result in severe sensations of dizziness. Visual disturbances can have either a central or peripheral origin. In order to differentiate between a central and peripheral visual impairment, the patient should be questioned as to whether they have double vision (diplopia), whether the visual disturbance becomes worse with head movement (i.e., VOR related), and whether there is any complete loss of vision. One of the most common forms of dizziness that occurs with neurological symptoms is migrainous vertigo. In fact, Isaacson and Rubin (1999) have reported that approximately one-third of the migraine population complains of associated vertigo. Tables 4–5 and 4–6 present otological and non-otological symptoms that can accompany dizziness, along with the potential causes.

Table 4–3. Common Disorders and Their Time Course

Short Duration	Intermediate Duration	Long Duration
BPPV Benign Paroxysmal Positional Vertigo	Migraine	Head injury (trauma)
Superior canal dehiscence	Metabolic disorders	Vestibular neuritis
Vascular insufficiency	Ménière disease	Stroke
Medication effects	Syphilis	Medication effects
Chiari malformation	Panic attacks	Labyrinthitis
	Transient ischemic accident	

Table 4–4. Characteristics of Vertigo and Potential Origin

Vertigo of Short Duration	Potential Origin
Change in the position of head or head and body	BPPV Benign Paroxysmal Positional Vertigo
Loud sounds or exertion	Superior canal dehiscence
Standing up or sitting up quickly	Orthostatic hypotension

Vertigo of Intermediate or Long Duration	Potential Origin
Stress	Anxiety and/or depression
Headache	Migraine or space-occupying lesions
Diet	Ménière disease
Upper respiratory infection	Vestibular neuritis/labyrinthitis
Head trauma	Concussion/blast exposure

Table 4–5. Otological Symptoms of Dizziness

Dizziness with Associated Otological Symptoms	Potential Causes
Tinnitus (non-pulsatile/pulsatile)	Ménière disease
	Acoustic neuroma
Hearing loss (conductive/sensory, neural/mixed)	Vestibular schwannoma
Fullness (pressure/popping)	Perilymph fistula
	Labyrinthitis
Otalgia	Cholesteotoma
Otorrhea	Stroke (anterior inferior cerebellar artery)
	Otitis externa
	Otitis media

Table 4–6. Neurological Symptoms of Dizziness

Dizziness with Associated Neurological Symptoms	Potential Causes
Headaches	Stroke
Weakness (paralysis/numbness)	Migraine
	Multiple sclerosis
Facial palsy	Vertebrobasilar insufficiency
Loss of consciousness	
Photophobia/phonophobia	Viral infection (Ramsay Hunt syndrome)
Dysphagia/dysphonia/dysarthria	Tumors
Changes in vision	
Ataxia	

Question 5: Do You Have Any Other Medical Conditions?

The patient's current medical status and medical history are important components in the case history because there are medical conditions that are known to contribute to dizziness. Prior to the face-to-face interview, the clinician should have reviewed the patient's medical history and noted any conditions that may indirectly or directly affect the vestibular system or contribute to sensations of dizziness. Any surgeries, otological or otherwise, should be documented and further examined. As with the associated symptoms, the patient can be questioned regarding any medical conditions that are otological or non-otological. For example, a patient who has a history of ear disease (e.g., cholesteotoma) may have had numerous surgeries, and based on the symptoms a causal relationship may be established. A patient who has heart disease (e.g., coronary artery disease) may likely complain of lightheadedness. In patients who are anxious or depressed, a relationship may exist between the dizziness and the situation that results in a patient having a panic attack. Finally, patients should be questioned regarding their family's history of neurological and/or otological disease. For example, questions inquiring whether there are any family members with migraine or multiple sclerosis can be helpful because many of the disorders that cause dizziness can be genetically transmitted. Table 4–7 shows common medical conditions and the symptoms of dizziness that they produce.

Question 6: What Medications Are You Taking?

The majority of patients seen for balance function testing are using medications to either treat dizziness or another medical condition. The examiner should have the patient bring a list of all prescription and over-the-counter medications (including nutritional supplements). It is the responsibility of the clinician to understand the symptoms and side effects that these medications have on dizziness and how these agents contribute to a patient's complaints. It is also important that the examiner be aware of the effect of medication on quantitative vestibular testing. Some medications affect the peripheral vestibular system, whereas others act on the central nervous system. Patients taking drugs that affect the nervous system may produce findings that are similar to those of patients with a cerebellar impairment, oculomotor impairment, or a decrease in peripheral vestibular system function. Patients suffering from an acute attack of vertigo are often prescribed antivertigo medications (meclizine or Valium). These medications act to reduce the symptoms of dizziness as well as prevent nausea and vomiting. To reduce the patient's

Table 4–7. Types of Dizziness and Related Medical Conditions

Medical Condition	Type of Dizziness
Cardiovascular	Syncope (orthostatic hypotension)
Migraine	Motion intolerance/ vertigo
Multiple sclerosis	Ataxia, lightheadedness, vertigo
Autoimmune disease	Ataxia, oscillopsia, lightheadedness
Chronic subjective dizziness	Rocking sensation, lightheadedness
Viral infections (nervous system)	Ataxia/vertigo
Stroke	Vertigo, short-duration unsteadiness

symptoms of vertigo, the actions of these medications work to target the neurotransmitters acetylcholine, histamine, and gamma-aminobutyric acid (GABA) at the level of the vestibular nerve and nuclei (Foster & Baloh, 1996; Baloh, 1998b). The antinausea mechanisms of the medications block the input to the medullary vomiting region and reduce the symptoms (Timmerman, 1994). The nature of these medications is such that they sedate the central nervous system and can thus produce abnormalities during oculomotor testing, static positional testing, and caloric testing. A summary of common medications and their effects is presented in Table 4–8.

ASSESSMENT OF DIZZINESS HANDICAP

Conventional tests of balance function (e.g., electronystagmography) yield valuable information regarding damage (impairment) to the balance system; however, these tests provide very little information regarding the debilitating effects

Table 4–8. Common Medications, Their Mechanisms, and Adverse Effects

Common Medications	Mechanism	Adverse Effect
Alcohol (e.g., Tennessee Moonshine)	Enhancement of GABA receptor function (global sedation of central nervous system)	Brainstem–cerebellar signs, positional nystagmus
Anticonvulsants (e.g., Dilantin[a], Tegretol[b])	Inhibits voltage-dependent sodium and calcium channels (thought to inhibit neuronal firing); enhancement of GABA receptor function	Brainstem–cerebellar signs, sedation
Antidepressants/anxiety benzodiazepines (e.g., Valium[c], Xanax[a])	Enhancement of GABA receptor function (global sedation of central nervous system including vestibular nerve and nuclei)	Brainstem–cerebellar signs, sedation, may inhibit central nervous system compensation, ataxia
Antivertigo/nausea antihistamines (e.g., meclizine)	Blocks dopamine (primarily inhibitory neurotransmitter) thereby increasing excitation at the level of the brainstem	Sedation, may inhibit central nervous system compensation
Aminoglycosides (e.g., vancomycin, streptomycin, gentamicin)	Act as protein synthesis inhibitors (disrupts bacteria growth)	Ototoxcity, neurotoxcity, vestibulotoxicity
Chemotherapeutics (e.g., cisplatin, carboplatin)	Acts as alkylating agents (inhibit cancer cells from growing)	Ototoxcity, neurotoxcity, vestibulotoxicity
Antihypertensives (e.g., Lasix[d], atenolol)	Diuretics diminish sodium reabsorption	Presyncope, orthostatic hypotension

[a]Pizfer, New York, N.Y.

[b]Novartis Pharmaceuticals, East Hanover, N.J.

[c]Roche Laboratories, Nutley, N.J.

[d]Sanofi Aventis, Bridewater, N.J.

GABA gamma-aminobutyric acid

(handicap) that disorders of the balance system may have on an individual's functional, emotional, and/or physical aspects of life (Jacobson & Newman, 1990). In this regard, the World Health Organization (WHO) has provided definitions to differentiate between impairment and handicap. The WHO defines "impairment" as an abnormality or loss of physiological, psychological, or anatomical structure or function (WHO, 2002). Using this definition, impairment in the balance system may be dysfunction in any of the systems necessary to maintain balance (i.e., vestibular system, visual system, and/or the proprioceptive system). Abnormalities of the balance system are often able to be confirmed through quantitative balance function tests (e.g., electronystagmography). Alterna-

tively, "handicap" is defined as a disadvantage for a given individual, resulting from an impairment that limits or prevents the fulfillment of a role that is normal" (WHO, 2002). In order for the clinician to obtain a complete picture of the patient's disability, an assessment of the patient's perceived handicap should be acquired. The challenge is that it is not uncommon for patients with a history of dizziness to be asymptomatic at the time of testing and therefore to have normal results on quantitative balance function tests. The clinician should be vigilant to the fact that sensations of dizziness and imbalance can lead the patient to restrict social and physical activities. Furthermore, patients experiencing dizziness may suffer from significant emotional distress that can be as debilitating as the symptoms of dizziness. It is imperative that the clinician keep in mind that each patient's response to the dizziness or imbalance is unique. In other words, the patient's reaction to the sensations vary based on their personality type, age, physical health, and/or psychosocial adjustment. Conventional balance function tests are incapable of assessing the degree of participation restriction and activity limitation caused by a balance disorder. To address this, Jacobson and Newman (1990) developed a measure known as the Dizziness Handicap Inventory (DHI).

The DHI is a 25-item questionnaire designed to assess the self-perceived handicapping effects of vestibular system disorders on patients. None of the items use the word "dizziness" but instead employ the term "problem" (Table 4–9). The DHI is grouped into three subscales: a 9-item functional scale, 9-item emotional scale, and 7-item physical scale. The functional scale was developed to assess what the effect of "the problem" is on the patient's daily life. The physical scale assesses how head and body movements affect "the problem," and finally, the emotional scale evaluates what effect "the problem" has on the patient's emotional well-being. Patients respond to each question by answering "yes," "sometimes," or "no" to each item and are given a score of 4, 2, or 0, respectively. Following completion of the scale, the examiner can calculate the score for each subscale or use the total score.

The DHI is a reliable and valid measure of the patient's perception of handicap (Enloe & Shields, 1997; Jacobson & Calder, 1998; Jacobson & Newman, 1990; Jacobson, Newman, Hunter, & Balzer, 1991). The total score of the DHI has good face validity and high internal consistency (Cronbach's alpha = 0.78–0.89) and high test–retest reliability ($r = 0.97$, $df = 12$, $p < 0.0001$). Satisfactory internal consistency was noted for the functional, emotional, and physical subscales ($\alpha = 0.72$–0.85). In an effort to describe the degree to which dizziness handicaps a patient's quality of life, Jacobson and McCaslin (unpublished data) categorized the level of severity using the total score of the DHI. Specifically, the interquartile ranges for the total DHI score were calculated using the scores from 200 consecutive patients reporting to a dizziness clinic. A score of 0–14 points was considered to represent no dizziness handicap. Total DHI scores of 15–26 were classified as mild handicap, and a score of 27–44 was considered moderate handicap.

Table 4–9. Dizziness Handicap Inventory

Instructions: The purpose of this questionnaire is to identify difficulties that you may be experiencing because of your dizziness or unsteadiness. Please answer "yes," "no," or "sometimes" to each question.

Answer each question as it pertains to your dizziness problem only.

	Yes (4)	Sometimes (2)	No (0)
P1. Does looking up increase your problem?			
E2. Because of your problem do you feel frustrated?			
F3. Because of your problem do you restrict your travel for business or recreation ?			
P4. Does walking down the aisle of a supermarket increase your problem?			
F5. Because of your problem do you have difficulty getting into or out of bed.			

Table 4–9. *continued*

	Yes (4)	Sometimes (2)	No (0)
F6. Does your problem significantly restrict your participation in social activities such as going out to dinner, going to the movies, dancing, or to parties?			
F7. Because of your problem do you have difficulty reading?			
P8. Does performing more ambitious activities like sports, dancing, household chores, such as sweeping or putting dishes away, increase your problem?			
E9. Because of your problem are you afraid to leave your home without having someone accompany you?			
E10. Because of your problem have you been embarrassed in front of others?			
P11. Do quick movements of your head increase your problem?			
F12. Because of your problem do you avoid heights?			
P13. Does turning over in bed increase your problem?			
F14. Because of your problem is it difficult for you to do strenuous housework or yardwork?			
E15. Because of your problem are you afraid people may think that you are intoxicated?			
P16. Because of your problem is it difficult for you to go for a walk by yourself?			
P17. Does walking down a sidewalk increase your problem?			
E18. Because of your problem is it difficult for you to concentrate?			
F19. Because of your problem is it difficult for you to walk around your house in the dark?			
E20. Because of your problem are you afraid to stay home alone?			
E21. Because of your problem do you feel handicapped?			
E22. Has your problem placed stress on your relationships with members of your family and friends?			
E23. Because of your problem are you depressed?			
F24. Does your problem interfere with your job or household responsibilities?			
P25. Does bending over increase your problem?			

FUNCTIONAL	EMOTIONAL	PHYSICAL	TOTAL SCORE

From Jacobson and Newman (1990)

A total DHI score of 44 or greater was classified as severe dizziness handicap (Table 4–10). In a similar attempt to categorize dizziness handicap using the total DHI score, Kinney, Sandridge, and Newman (1997) reported similar scores from a sample of 51 dizzy patients.

CHRONIC SUBJECTIVE DIZZINESS

The clinician seeing dizzy patients inevitably encounters patients who complain not of vertigo, but of a constant dizziness or "rocking." These patients may also have normal results on quantitative assessments of vestibular system impairment and neuroimaging. This pattern of symptoms and findings on quantitative assessments can be suggestive of an anxiety disorder. It is now known that there is a strong relationship between anxiety and dizziness (Ruckenstein & Staab, 2009). In fact, McKenna, Hallam, and Hinchcliffe (1991) reported that approximately 64% of dizzy patients seen in an audiology clinic also had an associated anxiety disorder. In line with these findings, Furman and Jacob (2001) found that the prevalence of psychiatric disorders in dizzy patients is higher than that found in the general population. In an article by Odman and Maire (2008), 80–93% of patients with chronic dizziness had a psychiatric disorder contributing significantly to their symptoms. When patients suffering from dizziness and anxiety are compared with patients with either dizziness or anxiety alone, they remain symptomatic for longer periods of time, have poorer treatment outcomes, and report increased handicap. In order to begin the process of correctly identifying and treating these patients, Staab and Ruckenstein (2005) have worked to replace the vague terms "space and motion discomfort" and "phobic postural vertigo" with the term chronic subjective dizziness (CSD).

CSD is defined using both the results of a neurotological examination and the presence of a specific set of physical symptoms. The physical symptoms include the persistent sensation (greater than 3 months) of non-vertiginous dizziness that may include lightheadedness, heavy headedness, or a feeling of imbalance that is not apparent to others (Staab & Ruckenstein, 2007). Other complaints, such as a hypersensitivity to motion, and worsening of symptoms in complex visual environments are also suggestive of CSD. Interestingly, the term anxiety is purposefully excluded from the core definition of CSD in order to avoid the premature assumption that the patient's dizziness is due to a psychiatric disorder. The primary age range of patients presenting with CSD is 40–50 years with the majority being female. CSD occurs in patients with and without otological (e.g., neuritis) or neurological disease (e.g., migraine). In this regard, Staab and Ruckenstein (2005) have devised a classification system consisting of three patterns of illness (Table 4–11).

Table 4–10. Dizziness Handicap Inventory Data

Quartile	Score	Handicap
1	0–14	None
2	15–26	Mild
3	27–44	Moderate
4	44+	Severe

From Jacobson and McCaslin (unpublished data)

Table 4–11. Types and Descriptions of Chronic Subjective Dizziness (*CSD*)

Type of CSD	Description
Otogenic	Patient without a prior history of anxiety disorder develops one after an acute vestibular impairment (i.e., otological illness precipitates the onset of anxiety)
Psychogenic	Patient with no history of physical disorders develops dizziness as part of their primary anxiety disorder
Interactive	Patient has a history of anxiety disorder before the onset of dizziness; develops CSD and a worsening of the anxiety disorder subsequent to vertigo (e.g., neuritis) or dizziness

The determination of whether a person has CSD or not is based on several factors which include a case history, self-report measures of anxiety/depression, dizziness handicap, and results of quantitative balance function testing (e.g., ENG/VNG). One instrument that has been employed to screen for the presence of anxiety and depression is the Hospital Anxiety and Depression Scale (HADS). The HADS is a 14-item self-report scale developed to detect anxiety and depression in a medical outpatient clinic (Zigmond & Snaith, 1983) (Table 4–12). The HADS has been reported to be a reliable measure for screening current states of anxiety and depression. The anxiety and depression subscales each consist of 7 items and each item is assigned a score from 0 to 3 points. For each of the subscales a score of 11 or greater is associated with the presence of clinically significant anxiety or depression (Zigmond & Snaith, 1983) (Table 4–13).

GROSS EYE MOVEMENT EXAMINATION

There are several reasons why the clinician should always perform an examination of the movement of the eyes before any formal testing begins. First, this brief examination provides valuable information regarding the integrity of the cranial nerves and central nervous system control of the eyes (i.e., saccades and gaze). Second, it reveals if the range of motion of the extraocular muscles (EOMs) is intact and the eye movements are conjugate (move together). Finally, a close evaluation of the eyes allows the examiner to identify the presence of any nystagmus. Having this information prior to performing the VNG enables the clinician to adapt the test protocol, if necessary, and avoid technical errors and misinterpretation of the examination. For instance, the clinician occasionally encounters patients presenting with abnormalities of the eyelid. One such abnormality is referred to as ptosis (Greek for *fall*). Ptosis is a drooping of one or both eyelids and is readily identified during the gross eye movement examination. Ptosis may be suggestive of impairment to the muscle that lifts the eyelid or impairment to the oculomotor nerve

(cranial nerve III) which controls the muscle or involvement of the superior cervical sympathetic ganglion. Bilateral and unilateral ptosis has also been associated with genetic disorders involving the oculomotor nerve (i.e., CFEOM1, CFEOM3, and congenital ptosis) (Leigh & Zee, 2011). When recording the eye movements of a patient with unilateral ptosis a monocular recording (of the intact eye) is often indicated.

For the purpose of reporting findings during the gross eye movement examination, it is important that the clinician understand the terminology that accompanies the descriptions of how the eye moves. For instance, a horizontal movement of an eye away from the nose is commonly referred to an A-B-duction, and a movement of the eye toward the nose is called an A-D-duction (Figure 4–1). When referring to movements in the vertical plane, an upward movement of the eye is known as an elevation and a downward movement is referred to as a depression.

The eye can also rotate, and these types of movements are described as torsional movements. There are two types of torsional eye movements. When the eye rotates toward the nose it is referred to as intorsion and when it rotates away from the nose it is called extorsion. There are two primary reasons that it is critical to identify when a patient does not have conjugate eye movements. First, when the clinician is preparing the patient for the ENG/VNG test, if the eyes are determined to not be conjugate, he or she needs to make sure that each eye is recorded from separately. Second, identifying disconjugate eye movements can provide insight into a patient's reported symptoms and impairment. For example, a patient with disconjugate eye movements often complains of double vision (diplopia). Diplopia is commonly observed in patients with either a mechanical problem affecting the EOMs, a lesion in the neuromuscular junction (brainstem), or a disorder affecting the cranial nerves that innervate the EOMs (oculomotor, abducens, or trochlear). An example of one such disorder is internuclear opthalmoplegia (INO). There are varying levels of severity of INO ranging anywhere from simply slow movements of the adducting eye (the eye moving toward the nose) to total paralysis. INO can be either unilateral or bilateral and implicates the medial longitudinal

Table 4–12. Hospital Anxiety and Depression Scale (HADS)

The purpose of this questionnaire is to identify feelings and emotion that you may be having. Each of the statements below gives an example of an emotion that may or may not apply to you. Do not analyze the statements in detail. Circle the answer that best fits your current situation.

1. I feel tense or wound up:
   a. Most of the time
   b. A lot of the time
   c. From time to time, occasionally
   d. Not at all

2. I still enjoy the things I used to enjoy:
   a. Definitely as much
   b. Not quite as much
   c. Only a little
   d. Hardly at all

3. I get a sort of frightened feeling as if something awful is about to happen:
   a. Very definitely and quite badly
   b. Yes, but not too badly
   c. A little, but it doesn't worry me
   d. Not at all

4. I can laugh and see the funny side of things
   a. As much as I always could
   b. Not quite as much now
   c. Definitely not so much now
   d. Not at all

5. Worrying thoughts go through my mind:
   a. A great deal of the time
   b. A lot of the time
   c. From time to time, but not too often
   d. Only occasionally

6. I feel cheerful:
   a. Not at all
   b. Not often
   c. Sometimes
   d. Most of the time

7. I can sit at ease and feel relaxed:
   a. Definitely
   b. Usually
   c. Not often
   d. Not at all

8. I feel as if I am slowed down:
   a. Nearly all the time
   b. Very often
   c. Sometimes
   d. Not at all

9. I get a sort of frightened feeling like"butterflies" in the stomach:
   a. Not at all
   b. Occasionally
   c. Quite often
   d. Very often

10. I have lost interest in my appearance:
    a. Definitely
    b. I don't take as much care as I should
    c. I may not take quite as much care.
    d. I take just as much care as ever

11. I feel restless as if I have to be on the move:
    a. Very much indeed
    b. Quite a lot
    c. Not very much
    d. Not at all

12. I look forward with enjoyment to things:
    a. As much as I ever did
    b. Rather less than I used to
    c. Definitely less than I used to
    d. Hardly at all

13. I get a sudden feeling of panic:
    a. Very often indeed
    b. Quite often
    c. Not very often
    d. Not at all

14. I can enjoy a good book or radio or TV program
    a. Often
    b. Sometimes
    c. Not often
    d. Very seldom

Modified from Zignond and Snaith (1983)

Table 4–13. Hospital Anxiety and Depression Scale (HADS) Scoring

Question Number	Item Answers A	B	C	D	Item Score
1					
3					
5					
7					
9					
11					
13					
Anxiety Score (sum from odd-numbered questions)					
2					
4					
6					
8					
10					
12					
14					
Depression Score (sum from even-numbered questions)					
Total Score (Anxiety + Depression)					

Modified from Staab (2008).

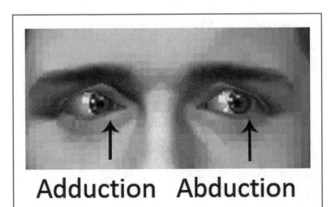

Adduction   Abduction

FIGURE 4–1. Image shows the adducting eye and abducting eye. Abduction is a horizontal movement of the eye away from the midline (*right arrow*). Adduction is a horizontal movement of the eye toward the midline (*left arrow*).

fasciculus (reviewed in Chapter 1). This disorder is commonly observed in patients suffering from multiple sclerosis or brainstem stroke. An INO should be identified prior to testing during the gross eye movement examination. Figure 4–2 illustrates the eye movements of a patient with an INO during the gaze examination.

The examiner should also note and describe any nystagmus observed during the gross eye movement examination. Nystagmus (described in Chapter 2) can be either physiological (i.e., normal) or pathological (i.e., abnormal) (Baloh, 1998a). Physiological nystagmus can be induced several different ways. For example, it can be observed when a patient is rotated in a chair, subjected to a full-field stimulus (optokinetic),

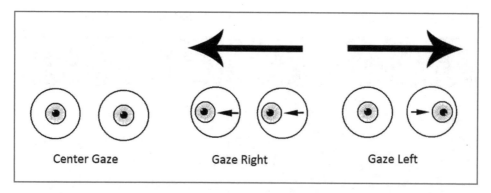

FIGURE 4–2. Illustration of the eye movements of a patient with right internuclear opthalmoplegia. The right eye is affected, and when gaze is directed to the left there is an impairment of adduction.

induced by a caloric stimulus into the ear canal, or stimulated when the eyes are driven to extremes during lateral gaze (i.e., greater than 40°). There also several varieties of pathological nystagmus. The three primary types are spontaneous, gaze evoked, and positional (Baloh & Kerber, 2011). When the examiner performs a gross eye movement evaluation he or she must be able to discern normal nystagmus from abnormal nystagmus. If it is determined that a patient has pathological nystagmus, the direction (e.g., down-beating or up-beating), effect of eye position (e.g., enhancement on lateral gaze), and effect of fixation should be described. One common method of describing the effect of eye position on nystagmus has been reported by Baloh and Honrubia (1990). This method makes use of a "tic-tac-toe" plot that represents the cardinal positions of gaze Arrows are drawn longer or shorter to represent the intensity of the nystagmus. The direction of the arrow describes which way the fast phase of the nystagmus is beating.

Common Types of Nystagmus Observed During the Gross Eye Movement Examination

Spontaneous Nystagmus of Peripheral Origin

The characteristics of spontaneous nystagmus of peripheral origin are: (a) horizontal-torsional nystagmus, (b) significant decrease in intensity with fixation, and (c) unidirectionality (follows Alexander's law). A summary of the features of spontaneous nystagmus are presented in Figure 4–3 using the box diagram method. (See Chapter 3 for a detailed account of these characteristics.)

Down-Beating Nystagmus of Central Origin

The characteristics of down-beating nystagmus of central origin are (a) little or no change in intensity with fixation, and (b) enhancement on lateral gaze. A summary of the features of down-beating nystagmus are presented in Figure 4–4 using the box diagram method. (See Chapter 5 for a detailed account of these characteristics.)

Symmetrical Gaze-Evoked Nystagmus

The characteristics of symmetrical gaze-evoked nystagmus are: (a) bidirectionality (left-beating on left gaze and right-beating on right gaze), (b) little or no change in intensity with fixation, and (c) high frequency and low amplitude. A summary of the features of gaze-evoked nystagmus are presented in Figure 4–5 using the box diagram method. (See Chapter 5 for a detailed account of these characteristics.)

Congenital Nystagmus

The characteristics of congenital nystagmus are: (a) conjugate high-frequency nystagmus, and (b) nystagmus that is variable in direction. A sum-

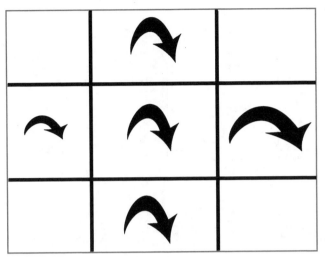

FIGURE 4–3. Example of how a left-beating peripherally generated spontaneous nystagmus that follows Alexander's law would be characterized using the method described by Baloh and Honrubia (1990).

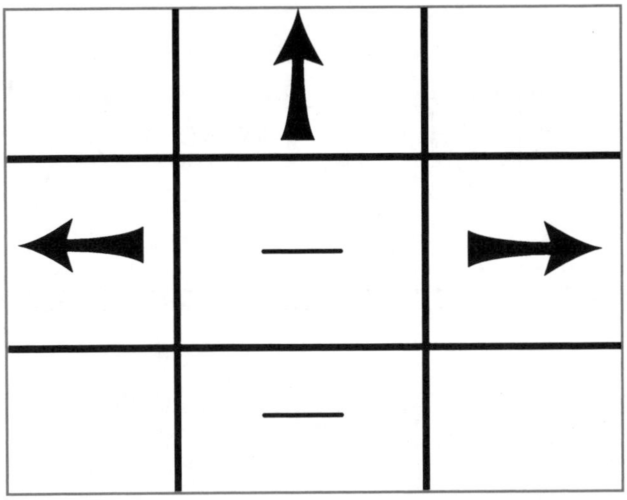

FIGURE 4–5. Example of how a bidirectional centrally generated gaze-evoked nystagmus would be characterized using the method described by Baloh and Honrubia (1990).

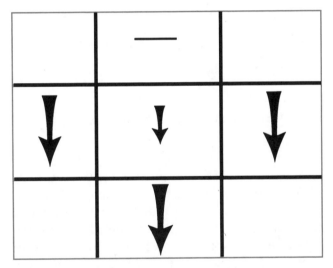

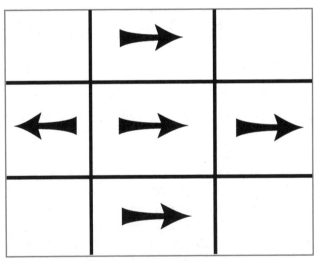

FIGURE 4–4. Example of how a down-beating centrally generated spontaneous nystagmus would be characterized using the method described by Baloh and Honrubia (1990).

FIGURE 4–6. Example of how a congenital nystagmus would be described using the method described by Baloh and Honrubia (1990). Note that on upward gaze the nystagmus continues to be horizontal.

mary of the features of congenital nystagmus are presented in Figure 4–6 using the box diagram method.

Congenital nystagmus (CN) is observed at birth or very shortly afterward. Patients with CN may have normal vision or may be visually impaired. This type of nystagmus is important to identify early during the ENG/VNG examina-

tion for two reasons. First, CN is due to a genetic (X-linked recessive or dominant trait) or developmental brain defect that may preclude the need for further testing (Gay et al., 1974). Second, the clinician needs to be prepared to account for these eye movements during the interpretation phase of the various ENG/VNG subtests. Figure 4–7 illustrates how congenital nystagmus manifests during

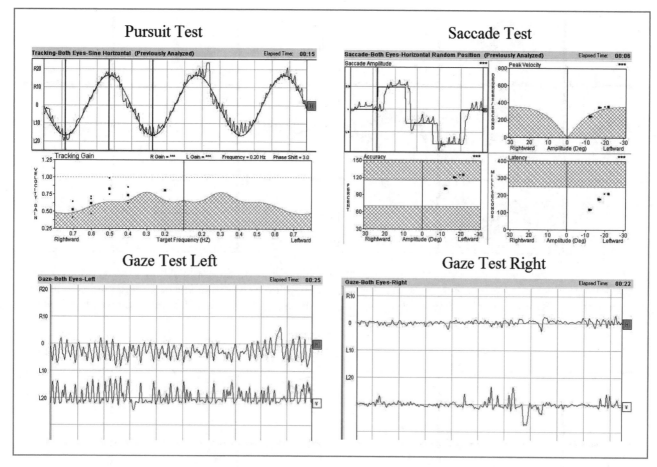

FIGURE 4–7. Example of how a congenital nystagmus manifests in various oculomotor subtests.

various oculomotor tests. CN is characterized by a bilateral pendular nystagmus or jerk nystagmus. The observed nystagmus is commonly conjugate and horizontal in all positions of gaze (including upward). Interestingly, patients do not complain of oscillopsia. This is important to note because it differentiates CN from nystagmus that is generated by brainstem or cerebellar impairments. The examiner, in some instances, may observe a small torsional or vertical component. When a patient with CN has his or her eyes near a certain orbital position, he or she has an eccentric neutral zone, or "null zone," where the nystagmus slows or is abolished. During converging eye movements CN nystagmus typically decreases. The decrease in CN intensity during convergence can be evaluated by having the patient fixate on a target 6 feet away and then bringing the target to 2 feet away. The intensity of the nystagmus should decrease or even stop. CN is more intense with arousal or visual attention, and CN may change direction with vision denied (e.g., during VNG). Finally, when the examiner is performing the gross eye movement examination it is a good practice to simply ask the patient "How long have your eyes moved that way?" The answer is typically "all my life."

Finally, the examiner should attend to how well the patient is able to follow instructions and sustain appropriate effort during the examination. This provides valuable insight into how well the patient will perform during the upcoming subtests of the ENG/VNG. Reinstruction should be provided if the patient has difficulty performing the task. In order to perform the gross eye movement examination, the examiner simply needs a chair, their fingers, and a pair of Frenzel glasses or VNG goggles.

Performing the Gross Eye Movement Examination

Instructions and Preparation

Seat the patient on the examination table in a room that is well lit and free of any moving distractions. Inquiry regarding the patient's visual acuity should be undertaken (e.g., glasses or prosthetic eye). A hand is placed on the patient's forehead to ensure that there will be no head movement. The patient should then be instructed to hold his or her head very still and follow the examiner's finger with his or her eyes.

Range of Motion

To evaluate the range of motion of the extraocular muscles, and whether the eyes are conjugate or not, the clinician draws a large imaginary "H" in the air (Figure 4–8). The legs of the H should be approximately 25–30° from midline. The vertical legs of the H pattern permit assessment of the inferior/superior oblique muscles and superior/inferior rectus muscles. The horizontal arm of the H tests the lateral and medial rectus muscles. The clinician should determine if

the patient's eye movements are conjugate (move identically).

Saccades

To evaluate the saccade system, the clinician should hold up each hand in a fist approximately 3 feet apart. The patient is then asked to quickly divert his or her gaze to the examiner's finger when it "pops" up, without moving the head. The clinician then proceeds to quickly lift an index finger on one hand at a time alternating left to right. The latency, accuracy, and velocity of the patient's eye movements should be observed.

Smooth Pursuit

To evaluate the smooth pursuit system, the clinician should place a hand on the patient's forehead to ensure that there will be no head movement. The patient should then be instructed to keep his or her head very still and follow the examiner's finger from side to side at approximately 2–4 Hz. The examiner should take care to note if the patient's eye movements are smooth and/or if they fall behind and then have to quickly catch up (saccadic pursuit).

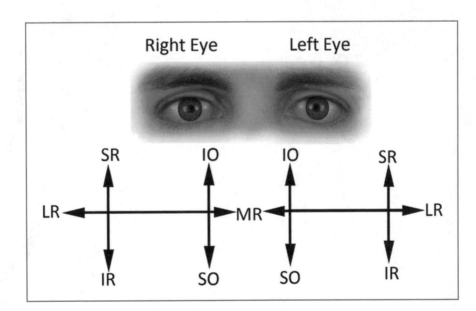

FIGURE 4–8. Movements of the extraocular muscles. **LR** lateral rectus; **SR** superior rectus; **IR** inferior rectus; **MR** medial rectus; **SO** superior oblique; **IO** inferior oblique; **SR** superior rectus. (Adapted from Nolan, 1996)

Gaze

To evaluate the gaze system the clinician should place a hand patient's forehead to ensure that there will be no head movement. The patient should then be instructed to keep their head very still and follow the examiner's finger approximately 30° up, down, right, and left. The examiner should take care to note any associated nystagmus and its characteristics (e.g., down-beating, up-beating).

Spontaneous Nystagmus

The last step in the gross eye movement examination is to evaluate the eyes with vision denied (e.g., VNG goggles with the shield down) or distorted (e.g., Frenzel glasses) while the patient is mentally tasked. A patient with Frenzel lenses is shown in Figure 4–9.

OTOSCOPIC EXAMINATION

Following an examination of the patient's eye movements, the clinician should inspect the external auditory canal and tympanic membrane in order to determine if any accommodations need to be made before the caloric examination. The ear canal should first be examined for any obstructing cerumen (Figure 4–10). In most ears there is some amount of wax. In cases where there is a cerumen impaction or enough wax that the clinician cannot see the tympanic membrane, the wax should be removed. A significant amount of wax can significantly impede the caloric stimulus and produce an erroneously reduced response. In cases where there is a significant amount of wax present, the

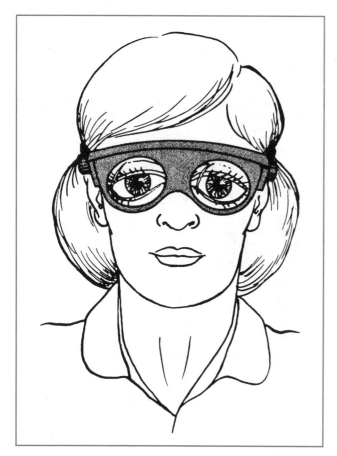

FIGURE 4–9. Illustration of a patient wearing Frenzel's lenses. (Illustration by Mary Dersch from Pender, 1992, with permission of Daniel Pender)

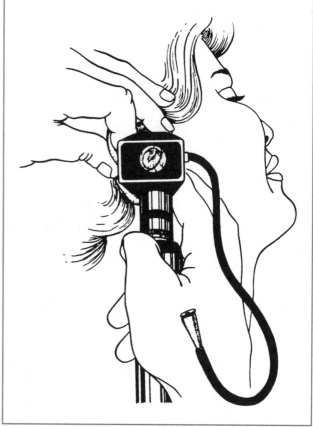

FIGURE 4–10. Illustration of a patient receiving an otoscopic examination. (Illustration by Mary Dersch from Pender, 1992, with permission of Daniel Pender)

examiner should prepare to remove the obstruction so that caloric testing can be performed. The clinician should also examine the ear canal for any anatomical anomalies that may affect caloric transmission. In cases of a surgical ear, caloric testing may be contraindicated. An otoscopic exam also provides the examiner with information about normal anatomical characteristics. For example, if the ear canals are tortuous, the clinician may need to retract the auricle and straighten out the ear canal in order to deliver an adequate caloric stimulus. After a careful inspection of the ear canal, the tympanic membrane should be examined. The clinician should be concerned with ensuring that the tympanic membranes are intact. If a perforation exists, then the use of water for generating the caloric response is contraindicated. In cases of tympanic membrane perforations, air can be employed as the stimulus; however, this can produce a caloric response that beats in a paradoxical direction and can be confusing to the clinician. A detailed account of what to look for during the otoscopic exam prior to the caloric exam is presented in Chapter 7.

THE VNG ENVIRONMENT

The VNG examination room should be large enough to accommodate the examiner, patient, and a person accompanying the patient. This environment should also be large enough to allow the clinician to move around freely. An ideal room for VNG testing is at least 10 feet wide and 14 feet long (Figure 4–11). These dimensions provide for enough room to have a sink, casework for the equipment to sit on, an examination table, and a stool for the examiner. Figure 4–11 shows the layout of a typical VNG examination room. Besides the dimensions, there are some key features that should be in the room. First, the room should have appropriate ventilation and a thermostat so that the room can be heated and cooled as needed. For example, in a hospital setting an inpatient may arrive at the appointment wearing only a gown, or in cases of patients with severe motion intolerance a cool room helps mitigate the effects of nausea. Another key feature is the ability to have nearly complete

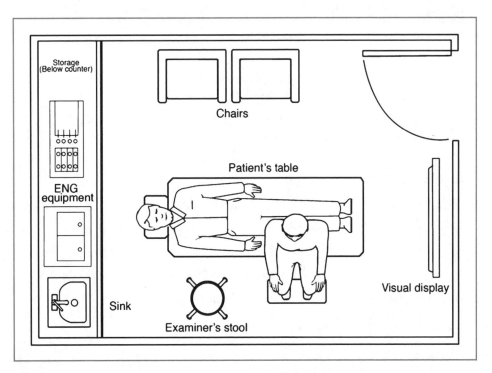

FIGURE 4–11. Illustration of a layout of a typical VNG laboratory.

darkness. Although most of the testing is done with dim light, there may be occurrences where it is desirable to have nearly complete absence of light (e.g., during the caloric testing or when there is a need to increase pupil size to help the VNG system track the eye). Table 4–14 shows equipment and Table 4–15 shows supplies that are required for the conventional ENG/VNG laboratory.

Table 4–14. Equipment Used in a Conventional ENG/VNG Laboratory

Equipment	Use
Examination table	Should be either a hydraulic or mechanical table that allows for positioning the patient anywhere from sitting to supine. An additional feature is the ability to remove the headrest for tests such as the Dix-Hallpike maneuver.
Caloric irrigator	Deliver caloric stimulus; can be air or water.
Recording system	Should be capable of measuring and recording eye movements using VNG or ENG.
Cabinet for supplies	Storage of supplies and patient-counseling materials.
Examination stool	For examiner to sit with patient and take case history and deliver caloric stimulus.
Visual stimulation system	Should be capable of producing appropriate stimuli for oculomotor testing (e.g., light bar or projector).

Table 4–15. Supplies Used in a Conventional ENG/VNG Laboratory

Supply	Use
Disposable electrodes	Recording EOG (when VNG is not indicated or cannot be performed).
Dental napkins	When using water caloric irrigations, these act to catch any water that may come out of the ear canal.
Paper pillowcases or disposable pillows	Provide comfort for those patients with neck or back impairments.
Alcohol, abrasive gel, gauze, cotton swabs	Preparing patient's skin for the recording of EOG.
Wax-removal tools	To remove cerumen in cases where the ear canal is blocked.
Irrigator specula or water-delivery tubes	Each patient should have their caloric irrigation delivered through a clean system.
Bleach	If using water, the baths should be bleached regularly.
Laboratory thermometer, graduated cylinder, and stopwatch	To calibrate water bath.
Emesis basins	Catch water when performing caloric or for use if patient becomes sick.

EOG = electro-oculography

5

Eye Movement Examination

INTRODUCTION

In order to evaluate the integrity of the peripheral vestibular system, clinicians must be able to do sophisticated recording for each of the different functional classes of eye movements. While it is difficult to obtain direct recordings from the peripheral vestibular system, the eye movement system affords the clinician a way to access the organs and nerves of balance via central nervous system connections located in the cerebellum and brainstem. Abnormalities identified during the eye movement examination can both provide the clinician with insight into the causes of a patient's reported dizziness as well as avoid misinterpretation of recordings obtained during the caloric test. A comprehensive clinical evaluation of the oculomotor system also provides valuable information for the referring physician to use during his or her differential diagnosis. Although a multitude of techniques exist for studying eye movements, this chapter describes only ENG and VNG.

INSTRUMENTATION

Eye Movement Recording Systems

The quantitative assessment of the oculomotor system and vestibulo-ocular reflex (VOR) is accomplished using either electro-oculographic (EOG) or video eye-tracking systems. Over the past decade there have been rapid advances in the quality and sensitivity of video eye-tracking systems. The majority of new systems sold in the United States now incorporate some form video eye-tracking technology (M. Petrack, personal communication).

Video Eye-Tracking Systems

Video eye-tracking systems employ specialized infrared cameras that can exploit the reflective properties of the corneal surface in order to calculate pupil position and angle of gaze. These cameras are typically mounted to either the top or side of a goggle system that is affixed to the head (Figure 5–1). An infrared illumination source that has the same orientation as the cameras is directed toward a mirror(s) composed of dichroic glass. Dichroic mirrors are simply glass that is coated with multiple layers of metal oxides that allow certain wavelengths of light to pass through (e.g., room light) or be reflected (e.g., infrared). Dichroic glass placed in front of the eyes at an angle enables the patient to look through the mirrors unobstructed while the infrared image of the eye is reflected to the cameras (Figure 5–2). The reflection of the eye that is received by the cameras is subjected to an analysis known as the "bright-pupil technique." This process causes the pupil to appear bright compared with the surrounding iris. The contrast between the iris and the pupil allows the video system to track the eye (Figure 5–3). This is accomplished by applying an algorithm that identifies either an elliptical portion of the pupil or the center of the pupil. In most systems the clinician is afforded the ability to focus and adjust the pupil/iris "brightness" for

maximum contrast. This ensures that the cross-hairs of the tracking system stay locked on the pupils as the eyes move.

EOG/ENG: CORNEORETINAL POTENTIAL

EOG/ENG is the eye movement technique that involves converting the bioelectrical signal of the corneoretinal potential (CRP) into an electrical form that can be collected and analyzed using a recording system. The eye has an electrical charge that is similar to a battery. In other words, the front of the eye (cornea) is positively charged while the back of the eye (retina) is negatively charged (Figure 5–4).

This dipolar electrical potential that exists between the retina and cornea of the CRP is maintained by metabolic activity in the retinal pigment epithelium (RPE). The RPE consists of a layer of hexagonal cells in the retina whose primary purpose is to protect the retina from excess incoming

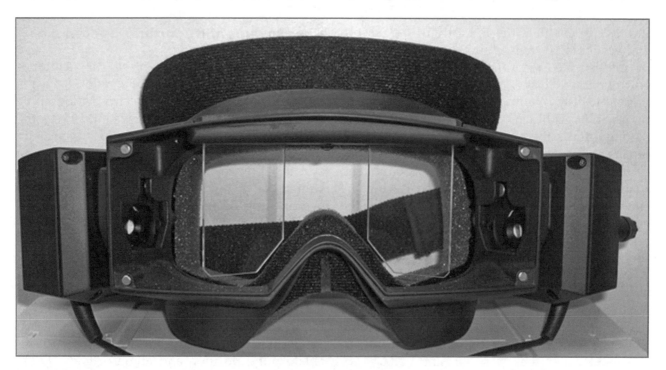

FIGURE 5–1. A binocular video eye movement recording system (Interacoustics, Assens, Denmark).

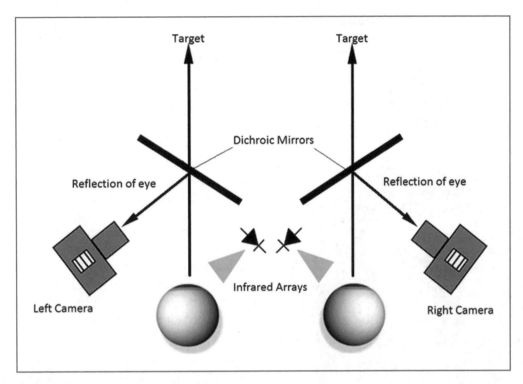

FIGURE 5–2. A basic illustration of the components and process of how a standard videonystagmography system operates.

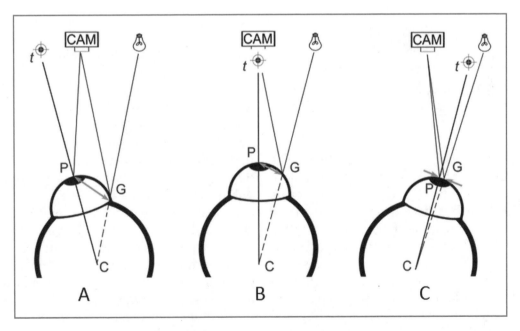

FIGURE 5–3. Bright-pupil oculography and the effects of movement of the eye on the magnitude of vector PG between the center of the pupil (*P*) and the center of the first Purkinje image (*G*). **A.** Movement away from the light source; **B.** eyes in the primary position; **C.** eye movement toward the light source. (From Jacobson, Shepard, Dundas, McCaslin, & Piker, 2008, p. 529)

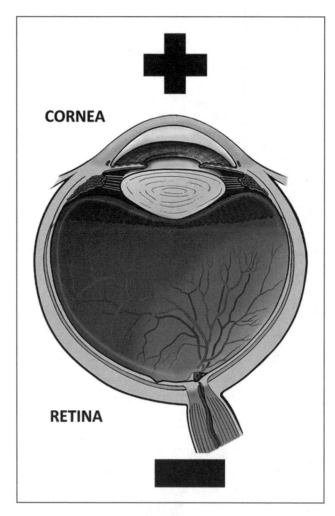

CORNEA

RETINA

FIGURE 5–4. The electrical potential between the cornea and retina is shown.

light (Carl, 1997; Marmor & Zrenner, 1993). The RPE cells are densely packed together enabling the eye to maintain its dipolar orientation or its CRP. The CRP is a dynamic potential and has been shown to vary across levels of illumination. When light enters the eye and falls on the RPE cells, the metabolic activity level in these cells increases. In this regard, if a patient is kept in a room with little or no light (dark adapted), the CRP potential will be smaller than if they were kept in a well-lighted room (light adapted).

Another factor has been reported to have a direct effect on the magnitude of the CRP. Some ENG systems allow the examiner to acquire an amplitude measurement of the CRP from the calibration data. According to Jacobson and McCaslin

(2004), there is a population of patients that generate "noisy" eye movement recordings when they are being tested using ENG (Figure 5–5). When the authors measured strength of the CRP in this subset of patients, it was found to be exceedingly low. In fact, the "noise" that was being recorded in the tracings was the noise floor of the amplifier. Jacobson and McCaslin (2004) went on to report that this group of patients with low CRP magnitudes also had retinal disease when they were evaluated by an ophthalmologist. In this regard, the strength of amplification of the CRP during calibration after the patient has been dark adapted could be a marker for retinal disease. Table 5–1 outlines the percentile values of the CRP for both men and women.

USING THE CRP TO RECORD EYE MOVEMENTS

Concept

The CRP can be used to track a patient's eye movements by placing electrodes on the outer canthi of the eyes. The process entails using differential amplification techniques to resolve the movement of the eyes. For example, in the case of a one-channel recording, if the non-inverting electrode is placed on the right side of the eye and the inverting electrode is placed on the left side of the eye, there is no voltage change while the eyes are in the primary position (Figure 5–6A); however, if the eye is moved to the right, the recording system will register an increase in voltage because the cornea (positive pole of the dipole) is being brought closer to the non-inverting electrode (Figure 5–6B). If the eye is deviated to the left, the cornea will be brought closer to the inverting electrode. In this case the increase in voltage will register as a decrease in voltage because the inverting electrode inverts the responses it records (positive becomes negative) (Figure 5–6C). This method is also employed to record vertical eye movements by placing a non-inverting electrode above the eye and an inverting electrode below the eye. When recorded in this fashion the magnitude of the CRP can range from 0 to 7 uV per degree of horizontal

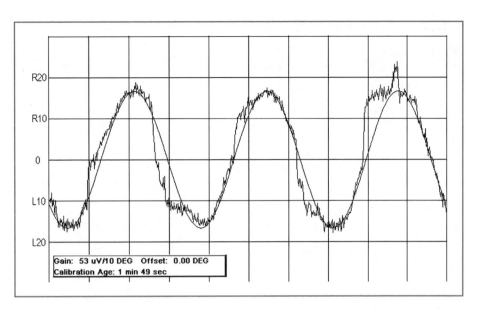

FIGURE 5–5. An ENG calibration in the horizontal plane obtained in an 80-year-old woman with advanced glaucoma and hypertensive retinopathy. (From Jacobson & McCaslin, 2004)

Table 5–1. Percentile Values Associated with Corneoretinal Potential Values Corresponding to 1° Eye Deviations from Midline

Sex	1st	5th	10th	15th	20th	50th	80th	85th	90th	95th	99th
M	7.1	8.2	9.2	9.5	10.4	13.8	17.3	19.1	19.9	21.8	25.8
F	9.0	10.8	11.4	13.0	13.2	17.2	21.7	22.2	24.5	27.3	28.2

Source: From Jacobson & McCaslin (2004)

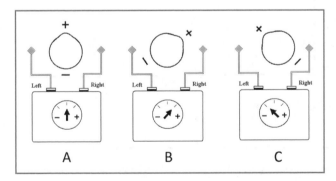

FIGURE 5–6. A–C. The corneoretinal potential and change in voltage registered at the electrodes with left and right eye movements. (From Jacobson et al., 2008, p. 28)

eye deviation (Jacobson & McCaslin, 2004). Table 5–2 provides a comparison between VNG and ENG recording techniques.

Clinical Application

When Eye Movements Are Conjugate

The determination of how many recording channels to use depends on whether the patient had full, conjugate range of motion of the eyes during the gross eye movement examination. In the majority of cases it is adequate to record the EOG using a "bitemporal" array. In this electrode montage a pair of electrodes (channel 1) is placed at the outer canthus of each eye. These electrodes are used to record lateral (right and left) eye movement and should be positioned so that if an imaginary line were drawn between them, it would pass through the center of the pupils. In order to record vertical eye movements a second pair of electrodes (channel 2) should be placed above and

Table 5–2. Comparison of VNG and ENG Recording Techniques

Variable	VOG/VNG	EOG/ENG
Spatial resolution	<0.5°	<1°
Vertical recording	Good (has capability to record and archive eye movements)	Occasionally interrupted by eye-blink artifact
Setup	Accomplished quickly	Takes longer than VOG due to electrode-preparation techniques
Cost	High cost	Low cost
Recording of torsional eye movements	Good	Poor
Effect of Bell's phenomenon[a]	None	Affected

VOG video-oculography; *EOG* electro-oculography

[a]Bell's phenomenon is an upward and outward reflexive movement of the eyes that occurs during eye closure. This reflex can cause induced nystagmus (e.g., produced during caloric or positional testing) to become dysrhythmic. This distortion can make interpretation of the response difficult when ENG is being used to record eye movements.

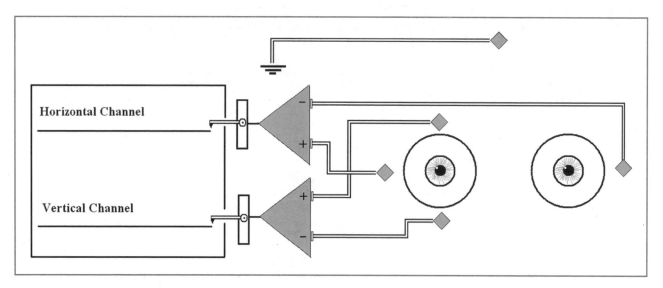

FIGURE 5–7. A bitemporal electrode montage and the connections to a two-channel differential amplifier electrode montage. (From Jacobson et al., 2008, p. 28)

below one of the eyes (Figure 5–7). The ground electrode should be placed on the forehead or nasion. A movement of the eyes to the right result in an upward deflection of the recording in the horizontal channel, whereas a movement of the eyes to the left creates a downward deflection in the same channel (Figure 5–8). For vertical eye movements, an upward movement of the eyes generates an upward deflection in the recording and a downward eye movement drives the record-

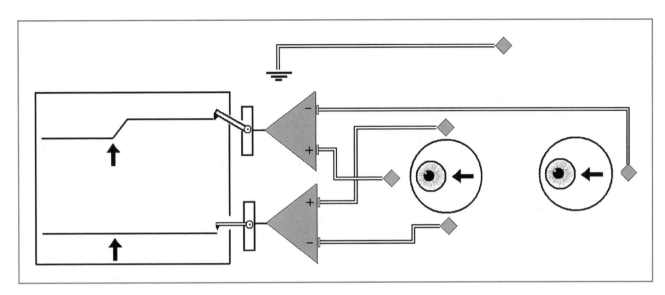

FIGURE 5–8. The horizontal and vertical amplifier outputs (*vertical arrows*) to a recording system for a rightward eye deviation (*horizontal arrows*). (From Jacobson et al., 2008, p. 28)

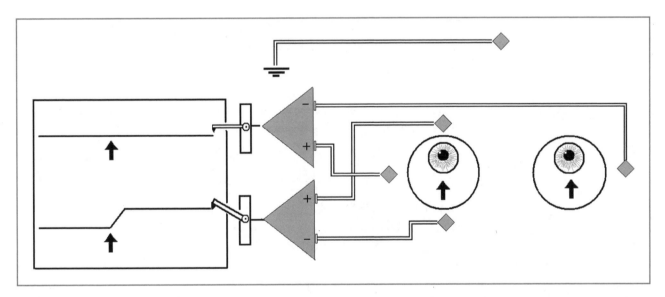

FIGURE 5–9. The horizontal and vertical amplifier outputs (*left arrows*) to a recording system for an upward eye deviation (*right arrows*). (From Jacobson et al., 2008, p. 28)

ing in a negative direction (Figure 5–9). Oblique eye movements change the voltage in both the vertical and horizontal channels at the same time (e.g., leftward and downward) (Figure 5–10). One of the limitations of recording with ENG is that the system is insensitive to purely torsional eye movements (e.g., counterclockwise or clockwise) (Figure 5–11).

When Eye Movements Are Not Conjugate

When a patient presents with disconjugate eye movements, the "bitemporal" recording method is not appropriate. This is because the CRP from each eye is averaged together when this electrode array is used. In cases where a patient presents with disconjugate eye movements, a monocular

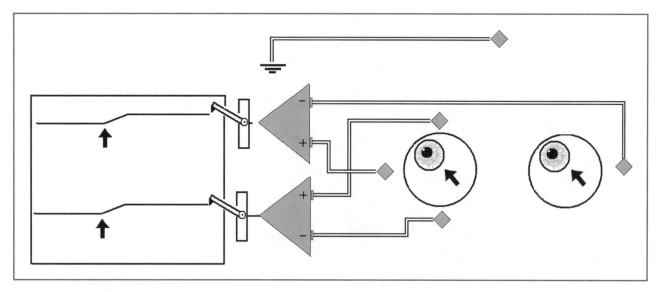

FIGURE 5–10. The horizontal and vertical amplifier outputs to a recording system for an oblique eye movement (*arrows*). (From Jacobson et al., 2008, p. 28)

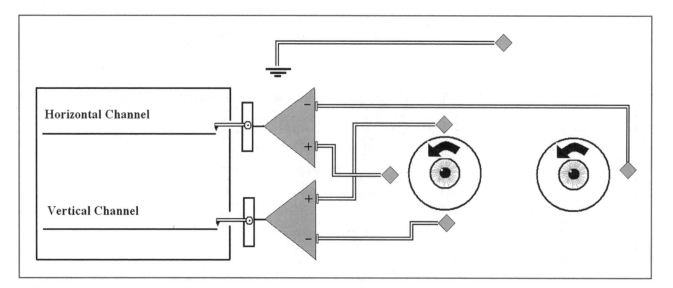

FIGURE 5–11. The horizontal and vertical amplifier outputs to a recording system for a completely torsional eye movement (*arrows*). (From Jacobson et al., 2008, p. 28)

electrode montage should be used. A monocular recording affords the clinician the ability to record the eye position of each eye separately. Figure 5–12 illustrates a four-channel recording that is capable of recording each eye independently. Each eye has a horizontal and vertical channel and the ground is placed on the forehead.

Calibration

The process of calibration involves converting eye movement into a digital representation that can be analyzed by the ENG/VNG computer. Early ENG systems recorded eye movement with red (vertical) and blue (horizontal) pens that would

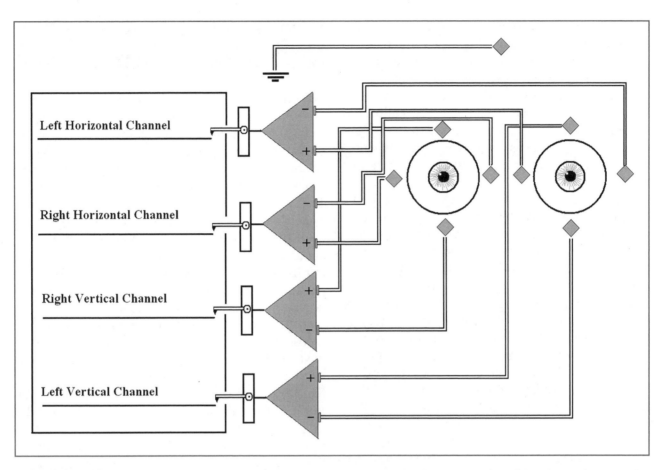

FIGURE 5–12. The horizontal and vertical amplifier outputs to a recording system for a four-channel monocular montage. (From Jacobson et al., 2008, p. 28)

transcribe the eye movement in the horizontal or vertical plane on a paper-strip chart (i.e., pen deflection). Most contemporary computerized ENG/VNG systems continue to display data in a similar way but in an electronic form. The calibration of an ENG/VNG system is based on the fact that the patient will be at a known distance from the visual stimulator. A common distance that manufactures use for the distance between the targets and the patient is 4 feet. Visual targets (e.g., lights) are placed in both the horizontal and vertical planes in such a way that an eye excursion of a person 4 feet away will be 10° from primary gaze (center gaze). To ensure that the patient is an appropriate distance from the target, some systems employ active range finders that let the examiner know whether the patient is too close

or too far. Once the calibration procedure is initiated and the patient acquires the target, the amplifier gain is adjusted so that the movement of the recording (horizontal and vertical) is equal in degrees to the eye movement (e.g., 10°). It is extremely important that the patient be the correct distance from the targets during the calibration process. If a patient is too close (less than 4 feet) or too far (greater than 4 feet), when the system is calibrated the conversion factor will be incorrect. For example, if a patient is 5 feet from the targets rather than 4 feet, the eye will move fewer than 10° (e.g., 6°) to acquire the target. The recording system will increase the gain to match the 6° eye movement to the target that is 10° from primary gaze. In this way the system overestimates the eye movement (e.g., a 6° eye movement is represented as a 10° eye movement). Alternatively, if the patient is only 3 feet from the target, the eye will need to move more than 20° to acquire the target (e.g., a 15° eye movement is represented as a 10° eye movement by the recording system). Data collected from an improperly calibrated system can lead to a misinterpretation (e.g., bilateral caloric weakness or hyperactive response) because of the over- or underestimation of the eye movements.

Whether the examiner uses ENG or VNG, the procedure for calibrating the system remains the same. What is different is the number of times that the ENG system must be recalibrated during the examination compared with the VNG system. Given that VNG goggles rely on tracking the pupil, as long as the goggles are not moved there is no need to recalibrate; however, as described in the previous section, ENG relies on the recording of the CRP, which is a dynamic electrical potential. The amplitude of the CRP varies depending on the amount of light in the environment. This is because the level of metabolic activity in the RPE changes depending on the level of illumination. On average, there is nearly a twofold increase in the amplitude of the CRP when an individual that has been dark adapted is moved to an illuminated environment and then light adapted (McCaslin & Jacobson, 2010). Lightfoot (2004) reported that approximately 6 to 9 minutes are required to fully light adapt an individual and 7 to 12 minutes to completely dark adapt. Accordingly, the recording system should be recalibrated approximately every 10 minutes until the CRP is stabilized, at which point the examiner should make every effort to ensure that the level of illumination is kept fairly constant for the duration of the test. A convenient time to calibrate is before the initial oculomotor subtest, again before positioning testing, and immediately before the first irrigation. While ANSI (1999) and BSA (1999) have recommended that the recording system be recalibrated prior to each caloric irrigation, it is the present author's opinion that this is unnecessary unless the level of illumination in the environment has changed, the electrodes have been moved, or there is an unexplained disagreement in the caloric responses.

SACCADE TEST

Saccade testing assesses specific structures in both the brainstem and cerebellum used to initiate saccades (see Chapter 1 for a detailed review). In the beginning, the assessment of saccades was accomplished with the examiner asking the patient to look at small dots fixed to the wall or ceiling. Today's computerized systems utilize projection systems and light bars and can present targets in a multitude of ways. Targets can now be presented at fixed and randomized times and locations. During the randomized paradigm, visual stimuli are presented in unpredictable locations in both the horizontal and vertical plane, and the patient's ability to acquire the targets is measured. When assessing saccadic function, the randomization of stimuli has been suggested to increase the sensitivity of the test to disorders compared with a fixed protocol (Isotalo, Pyykkö, Juhola, & Aalto, 1995). Currently, the randomized paradigm is the most common presentation for evaluating the saccade subsystem during ENG/VNG testing and is the focus of this section. Figure 5–13 illustrates eye recordings taken in a patient during the presentation of stimuli using a random saccade paradigm.

Assessment of Saccades

The procedure for the saccade test is as follows:

1. Perform a gross eye movement examination to determine whether the eye movements are disconjugate or conjugate.
2. Calibrate the patient using either individual eye recordings (if disconjugate eye movements were observed) or both eyes averaged together (if conjugate eye movements were observed).
3. Instruct the patient carefully (e.g., "Do not move your head and try not to anticipate where the target is going to show up next").
4. Record the patient's saccades using a pseudorandom presentation where the targets are presented between 5 and 40° from midline with a fixed interstimulus interval.

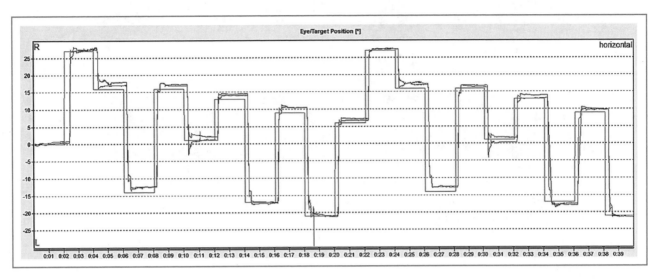

FIGURE 5–13. A recording of eye movements in response to a pseudorandom saccade paradigm.

5. Record and observe the eye movements for a duration that is sufficient to collect several patient responses for each saccade deviation (e.g., 30 s).
6. Analyze and inspect the data.
7. If abnormalities are noted, record for additional amount of time until it is confirmed that the abnormalities observed are repeatable and consistent (e.g., 30–50% of the responses are consistently abnormal).

Interpretation and Analysis

The three primary parameters that are used for the clinical analysis of saccades are how close the eye comes to acquiring the target (accuracy), the speed at which the eye moves to acquire the target (velocity), and the time it takes for the eye to move following a movement of the target (latency).

The sections below provide definitions of the analysis parameters and summaries of the causes of abnormality.

Accuracy

Accuracy describes how far over or under the target the eye was following its excursion to the target. If the eye falls significantly short of the target,

it is referred to as a hypometric response, and if the eye travels significantly past the target, it is hypermetric. A normal saccadic tracing with accuracy within normal limits is presented in Figure 5–14.

Velocity

Velocity refers to how fast the eye moves toward the target once the saccade has been initiated. Most systems calculate the peak eye velocity, which is the maximum velocity reached during the eye movement. It is noteworthy that the farther the target is away from the midline (e.g., 5 versus 35°), the higher the velocity must be for a response to be normal. This is because the eye movement system must overcome the viscoelastic forces that would normally keep the eyes in a neutral position. Once these forces have been overcome (i.e., as the eye moves further away from its starting point), the eye velocity increases. A normal saccadic velocity tracing is presented in Figure 5–15.

Latency

Latency reflects the difference in time (in milliseconds) between the presentation of a target and the initiation of the eye movement intended to acquire that target. A normal saccadic latency tracing is presented in Figure 5–16.

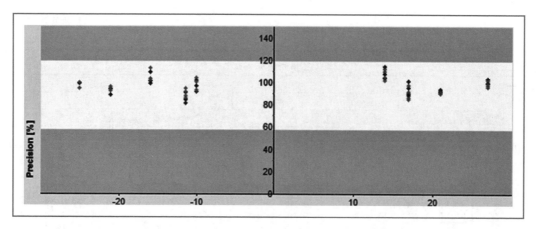

FIGURE 5–14. Saccade test accuracy data obtained in a normal individual. *Shaded* areas indicate abnormal accuracy.

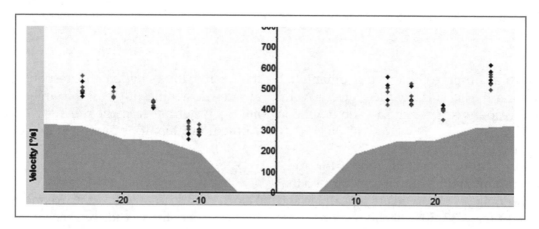

FIGURE 5–15. Saccade test velocity data obtained in a normal individual. *Shaded areas* indicate abnormally low velocity for a given target.

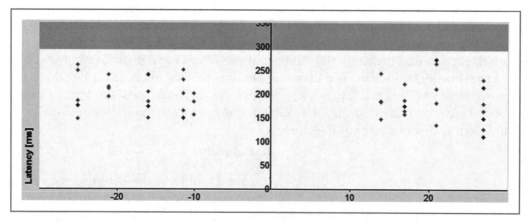

FIGURE 5–16. Saccade test latency data obtained in a normal individual. *Shaded areas* indicate abnormally long latency for a given target.

Saccade Abnormalities

As described in Chapter 1, a patient with impairment in the saccade eye movement system is unable to rapidly and accurately acquire a visual target or hold the eye on the target. This almost always involves abnormality of the pulse or step response (see Chapter 1 for a review).

The sections below provide descriptions of some common saccade disorders, cases illustrating these disorders, and a summary of each disorder's basic characteristics.

Velocity

Slow Saccades. Disorders of saccadic velocity involve a disorder in the pulse. The height of the pulse can be too big or too small, and the duration (width) can be too long or too short. The velocity of the saccade can also be asymmetric (each eye moves at a different speed). Abnormalities in the height and/or duration of the saccadic pulse affects the velocity of the eye when measured at the target. While the velocity of saccades is in large part controlled by burst neurons located in the paramedian pontine reticular formation (PPRF) or medial longitudinal fasciculus (MLF), the superior colliculus and cortex have also been shown to contribute (Leigh & Zee, 2006). Disorders that can result in a patient having slow saccades are basal ganglia syndromes, cerebellar syndromes, peripheral oculomotor nerve or muscle weakness, and white matter diseases. One classic example of a disorder that can cause saccadic slowing is internuclear opthalmoplegia (INO). There are varying levels of severity of INO ranging from simply slow movements of the adducting eye (the eye moving toward the nose) to total paralysis (Figure 5–17). INO can be either unilateral or bilateral and implicates impairment in the MLF (Leigh & Zee, 2006). Patients with a bilateral INO typically present with abducting nystagmus accompanied by weakness in the adducting eye. This disorder is typically observed in patients suffering from brainstem stroke. An INO should be able to be identified prior to testing during the gross eye movement examination and case history. While the majority of patients with an INO do not complain of dizziness, some may report double vision or even oscillopsia (Leigh & Zee, 2006). When abnormally low-velocity saccades are observed in a patient, the examiner must first rule out the contribution of medication and/or lack of alertness (Figure 5–18).

Fast Saccades. Patients can also present with abnormally high-velocity saccades. The causes of fast saccades can be a result of a mass or trauma to the eye, cerebellar impairments, and brainstem impairments. Calibration error should always be an initial consideration in patients who generate saccades that are too fast. If a patient continues to

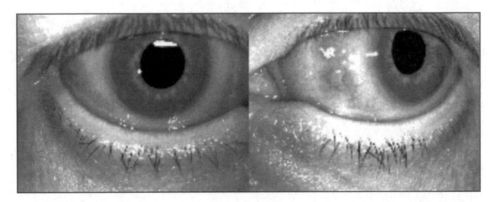

FIGURE 5–17. A patient with a right internuclear opthalmoplegia demonstrates impaired adduction of the right eye. The target is located 30° to the left from primary gaze.

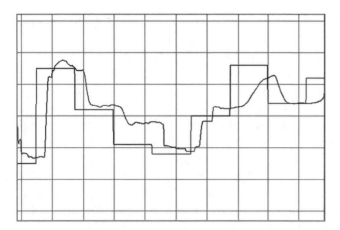

FIGURE 5–18. A recording of saccades in a patient who was heavily medicated and extremely drowsy at the time of testing.

generate abnormally fast saccades following recalibration, the clinician should check whether the saccades are of normal amplitude and whether the patient has full range of motion for both eyes. The velocity of the eye during a saccade is proportional to the distance the eye must travel. In other words, the eye generates higher-velocity movements for targets farther away and slower-velocity movements for targets that are closer. In cases where the eye has a restricted range of movement, the eye may be stopped before it reaches the target. According to Leigh and Zee (2006), the central nervous system calculates the size of the pulse based on the eye's position relative to the target. If the eye is stopped prematurely during the saccade, an analysis of the waveform will suggest that the velocity is abnormally high. This is because prior to the eye being halted, it was traveling at a velocity calculated to acquire a target further away (required a higher velocity); however, because the eyes are stopped short of the target, the amplitude of the saccade is lower than normal for the target.

Accuracy

Saccadic Pulse Dysmetria. Another type of saccade abnormality is called saccadic pulse dysmetria. The cerebellar vermis is responsible primarily for the accuracy of saccades. When damaged, the cerebellum cannot correctly calculate the amplitude of the saccade that is needed to acquire the target. The pulse (velocity signal) of the saccadic pulse-step step system is defective, causing the patient to overshoot (hypermetric) or undershoot (hypometric) the visual stimulus. When the saccade is too large or too small, a corrective saccade is generated to bring the eye onto the target.

In the case of a hypermetric saccade, the eye has overshot the target and must be moved in the direction opposite the target. The main characteristic of hypermetric saccades is that the eyes overshoot the target, remain at a fixed point a few degrees beyond the target for approximately 150–200 ms, and then return to fixate on the target. The mechanism is incorrect calculation of what the pulse-step should be by the neural integrator. These findings are suggestive of an impairment in the cerebellar dorsal vermis. Whenever hypermetric saccades are observed, caution should be exercised to rule out a visual impairment (e.g., macular degeneration), blinking, and improper calibration. (Note that over- or undershoots must be repeatable and consistent. If the patient generates normal saccades with only occasional over- or undershoots, the test is interpreted as normal.) Figure 5–19 illustrates the recordings from a patient with bilaterally hypermetric (overshoots) saccades. The recordings show that the eyes consistently pass by the target (overshoot) but then quickly return to fixate on the target.

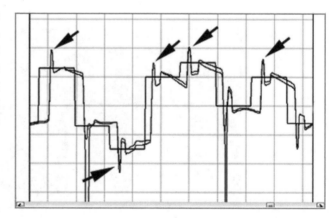

FIGURE 5–19. Hypermetric saccades (i.e., overshoots; *arrows*) generated by a patient with a cerebellar impairment.

The main characteristic of hypometric saccades is that the eyes undershoot the target, remain at a fixed point a few degrees short of the target, and then move again to acquire the target. Hypometric saccades can be either unidirectional or bidirectional. Causes of hypometric saccades include cerebellar impairments, internuclear ophthalmoplegia, supranuclear palsy, and basal ganglia disorders. Whenever hypometric saccades are recorded, caution should be exercised to rule out a visual impairment (e.g., macular degeneration), fatigue, medication, lack of alertness, and blinking. Figure 5–20 presents the eye recordings of a patient with consistent hypometric saccades.

Latency

Late Initiation of Saccades

Saccades can be initiated abnormally late (i.e., when the target moves to a new location, the eye has a prolonged latency before it starts to move); however, due to a vast number of pitfalls, latency is a relatively insensitive measure of saccade dysfunction when employed during the ENG/VNG battery. Factors affecting latency include age, lack of alertness, and inattention. Visual impairment has also been reported as a contributor to abnormally prolonged saccadic latency (Ciuffreda, Kenyon, & Stark, 1978). It is noteworthy that the abnormally prolonged initiation of saccades has been observed in patients with degenerative disorders (Fletcher & Sharpe, 1986; Leigh & Zee, 2006).

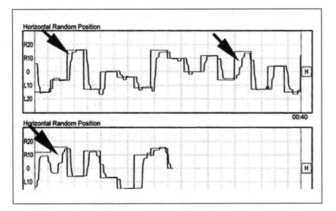

FIGURE 5–20. Hypometric saccades (i.e., undershoots; *arrows*) generated by a patient with a brainstem impairment.

GAZE TEST

The assessment of gaze involves evaluating the structures that are involved in fixation (see Chapter 1 for a review). In other words, the test is designed to determine if there is any aberrant nystagmus with the head oriented in the midline and the eyes at center position and looking horizontally and vertically. The gaze test is one of the most informative oculomotor tests but can also be one of the most difficult to interpret. This is because impairments in gaze stabilization can stem from peripheral abnormalities, central abnormalities, or both simultaneously. The primary feature that the examiner should be looking for when conducting the gaze-stabilization test is nystagmus. If nystagmus is present, the challenge for the clinician is to determine its origin.

The following two sections provide the recommended assessment techniques for gaze stabilization and how to interpret and differentiate central from peripheral involvement.

Assessment of Spontaneous Peripheral Nystagmus

Spontaneous peripheral nystagmus should be assessed in the following manner:

1. Instruct the patient to keep the head midline and fixate on the target (remember to reinstruct the patient to not move their head). The patient should be in the sitting position.
2. Record the eye movements for at least 30 s while tasking the patient.
3. Occlude vision and continue recording for at least another 30 s.
4. If nystagmus is observed, restore vision (or turn on a fixation light) and have the patient fixate on a target.

5. Record any changes in the nystagmus (reduction or increase in amplitude).

Assessment of Centrally Mediated Gaze-Evoked Nystagmus

Gaze-evoked nystagmus (GEN), which refers to nystagmus that increases in intensity as the eyes are brought from primary gaze position to eccentric gaze, should be assessed in the following manner:

1. Continue to have the patient keep the head midline and fixate on the target (remember to reinstruct the patient not to move their head). The patient should be in the sitting position.
2. Record at least 30 s of eye movement using targets placed at 30° from primary position (with vision present) for each of the subsequent gaze positions.
3. If nystagmus is found to be present, perform the test again to confirm that it is consistent. Additionally, the examiner should search for rebound nystagmus. Test sequence:
   a. Center gaze with eyes on target
   b. Center gaze with vision denied
   c. Right gaze with eyes on target (30°)
   d. Left gaze with eyes on target (30°)
   e. Up gaze with eyes on target (30°)
   f. Down gaze with eyes on target (30°)
4. If nystagmus is noted in any condition, repeat the examination until it is determined that the findings are consistent.

Interpretation and Analysis

When nystagmus is identified during any of the eye positions in the above sequences, there are three primary questions that must be answered in order to provide an accurate interpretation. First, in what direction does the nystagmus beat? Second, how does the intensity of the nystagmus change with visual fixation? Third, in what positions does the nystagmus occur? Answering these three questions correctly is critical for interpreting the gaze test and allows the examiner determine if the origin of the nystagmus is caused by a peripheral vestibular system impairment, a central eye movement system impairment, or both (Table 5–3).

Centrally Mediated Abnormalities in Gaze

Gaze-evoked nystagmus generated by central nervous system impairments can take many forms (e.g., vertical, oblique, horizontal). The nystagmus can vary in intensity and direction and can be bidirectional (right-beating on right gaze and left-beating on left gaze), down-beating, up-beating, or alternating.

Bilateral Gaze-Evoked Nystagmus

Significant GEN has been suggested to be nystagmus that is persistent during eccentric gaze of 30° or less (Hain, 1992). The main characteristic of bilateral GEN is small-amplitude nystagmus that is equal in intensity in all directions and observable when the eye is gazing eccentrically. The quick phase of the nystagmus beats away from the primary gaze position and is not suppressed by visual fixation. The causes of bilateral GEN are congenital nystagmus, and lesions in the cerebellum and/or brainstem. Bilateral GEN can also be caused by medications (anticonvulsants or sedatives) and/or alcohol.

The presence of GEN is often associated with a defect in the pulse-step relationship (described in Chapter 1). In other words, the burst neurons in the brainstem must generate an appropriate pulse to overcome the elastic restoring forces of the eye and bring the fovea to rest on the target. Once the eye reaches the target, neurons in the cerebellum and brainstem (i.e., neural integrator) generate a neural command to continually contract the extraocular eye muscles and hold the eye on the target (Leigh & Zee, 2006). This tonic response that keeps the eye from returning to its midline position is referred to as the step response (Leigh & Zee, 2006). Impairment in the neural integrator sets up a situation where the step response is inadequate and the eye slowly drifts off the target in the direction of primary gaze. Leigh and Zee (2006) have referred to this a "leaky" neural inte-

Table 5–3. Differentiation Between Central- and Peripheral-Gaze Nystagmus

What Is the Direction of Nystagmus?	
Peripheral	**Central**
Direction-fixed horizontal nystagmus	Direction changing in one or more gaze positions
Primarily horizontal with a slight torsional component	Direction fixed but purely vertical (up-beating or down-beating)
	Demonstrates rebound nystagmus (i.e., the direction of the nystagmus is always in the last direction that the eye moved)

What Is the Effect of Visual Fixation?	
Peripheral	**Central**
Enhanced intensity with vision occluded (i.e., vision denied)	Is present or enhanced with fixation
Diminished intensity with fixation invoked	Intensity does not change significantly with *removal* of fixation

In What Positions Does the Nystagmus Occur?		
	Primary Position	**Eccentric Gaze**
Peripheral	Horizontal nystagmus with a slight torsional component	Follows Alexander's law (i.e., horizontal nystagmus amplitude increases when the patient gazes in the direction of the fast phase; amplitude decreases when the patient gazes in the direction of the slow phase)
Central	Horizontal nystagmus (rarely observed in primary position)	Horizontal nystagmus observed (typically bidirectional (right-beating on right gaze and left-beating on left gaze)
	Vertical nystagmus (can be present in primary position)	Vertical nystagmus observed (typically enhances with vision)

grator (Figure 5–21). Once the oculomotor system detects that the fovea is no longer on the target, a saccade is generated in the direction of the gaze to reacquire the target. This pattern of the slow centripetal drift of the eye off the target followed by a saccade is the pattern of eye movement that is referred to as GEN (Figure 5–22). The clinician should be vigilant to the fact that GEN manifests during other tests of oculomotor function requiring eccentric gaze (Figure 5–23). Patients with bidirectional GEN often generate rebound nystagmus. Rebound nystagmus is an aberrant form of nystagmus that is observed in patients with brainstem and cerebellar diseases (Hain & Rudisill, 2008; Lin & Young, 1999). When the patient's eyes are brought back to midline from eccentric gaze, a brief (5 s) burst of nystagmus beating in the opposite direction of that in which the eye was gazing may be observed. For example, if the nystagmus is beating in the direction of eccentric gaze (e.g., right-beating on gaze right), when the eyes are brought back to midline, the nystagmus will beat to the left. If the nystagmus is left-beating on leftward gaze, when the eyes are brought back

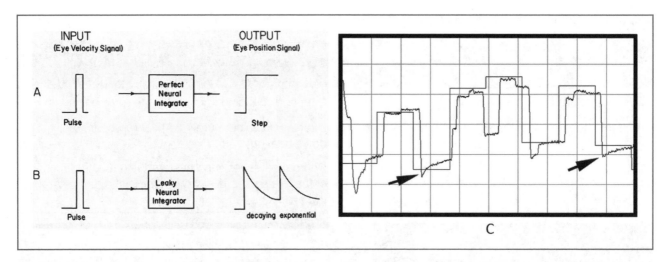

FIGURE 5–21. A–C. A simplified illustration of the neural integrator. **A.** A normal eye velocity signal (burst) and normal eye position signal (step response). **B.** A leaky neural integrator causes the eye position signal to decay. **C.** Recordings from a patient with a cerebellar impairment. The *arrows* designate where the eye begins to drift off the target due to an inadequate step response. (A and B from Leigh & Zee, 2006)

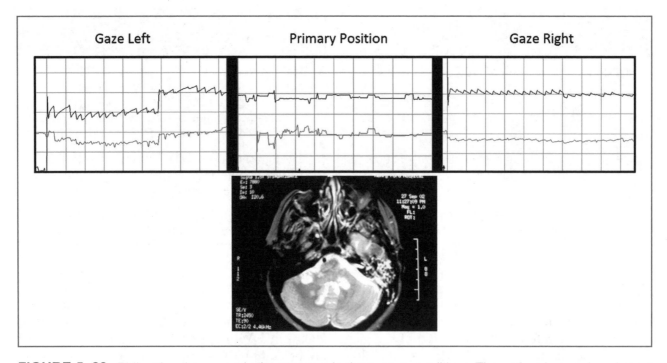

FIGURE 5–22. Bidirectional gaze-evoked nystagmus in three gaze conditions. The patient has an impairment affecting the cerebellum (i.e., multiple sclerosis).

to midline the nystagmus will be right-beating (Figure 5–24).

It is also important that the clinician distinguish between pathological GEN and a normal phenomenon known and "end-point" nystagmus. This type of nystagmus is occasionally observed in neurologically intact patients during extreme lateral gaze (e.g., >40°) (Figure 5–25). This form of nystagmus is low frequency and low amplitude, intermittent, and accompanies an otherwise normal oculomotor examination (Leigh & Zee, 2006. The nystagmus typically occurs immediately after moving the eyes to the eccentric position.

Down-Beating Nystagmus

Down-beating nystagmus is primarily vertical and enhances in intensity on eccentric gaze. It may or

may not be observed in the primary gaze position, but it commonly enhances on lateral or downward gaze (Figure 5–26). It is characterized by the fast phase of the nystagmus beating downward. Visual fixation does not suppress it significantly and the slow phases may increase or decrease in intensity. Patients with down-beating nystagmus often complain of oscillopsia or severe unsteadiness (retinal slip caused by the slow phase) (Leigh & Zee, 1991). The involvement of the cerebellum

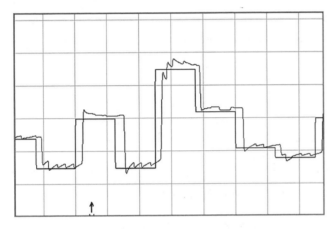

FIGURE 5–23. An example of how gaze-evoked nystagmus can be observed during other tests of ocular motility. In this case, bidirectional gaze-evoked nystagmus was observed during the saccade test.

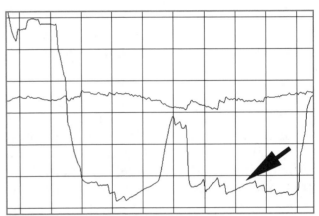

FIGURE 5–25. End-point nystagmus is shown (*arrow*).

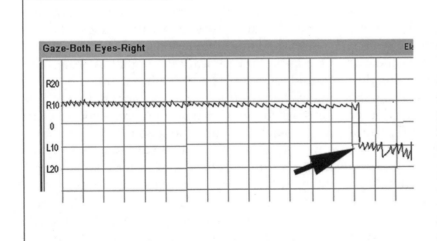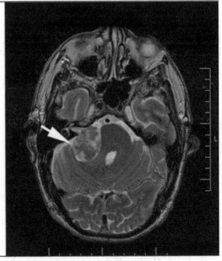

FIGURE 5–24. Rebound nystagmus in a patient with an impairment affecting the cerebellum. The *arrow* indicates the point where right-beating nystagmus shifts to left-beating nystagmus when the eyes move from right gaze to center gaze.

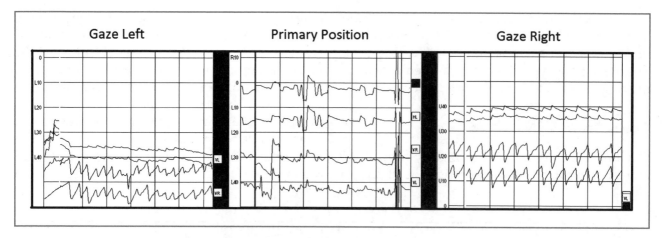

Gaze Left   **Primary Position**   **Gaze Right**

FIGURE 5–26. Down-beating nystagmus in different positions of gaze recorded in a 50-year-old patient diagnosed with midline cerebellar dysfunction (paraneoplastic).

also leads the patient to complain of postural instability and generalized imbalance. The presence of down-beating nystagmus implicates the vestibulocerebellum and medullary region of the brain and their connections to the semicircular canals (Leigh & Zee, 2006). Specifically, the cerebellum (i.e., flocculus) inhibits responses from the anterior semicircular canal (produces slow upward eye movements) but not responses from the posterior semicircular canal (produces slow downward eye movements) (Ito, Nisimaru, & Yamamoto, 1977; Baloh & Spooner, 1981). Because the vertical canals are paired (RALP and LARP), a loss of the inhibitory input to the anterior canals due to a cerebellar impairment causes the eye to slowly drift upward. The oculomotor system generates a downward saccade to reset the eye resulting in the pattern that is down-beating nystagmus. Figure 5–27 provides a diagram that illustrates one of the proposed origins of down-beating nystagmus (Ito et al., 1977; Baloh & Spooner, 1981). Down-beating nystagmus has been reported to be enhanced when patients are subjected to a "head-hanging" position (e.g., the Dix-Hallpike maneuver) (Marti, Palla, & Straumann, 2002). In this regard, care should be taken during the examination to not confuse down-beating nystagmus of central origin with benign paroxysmal positional vertigo (peripheral origin). The causes of down-beating nystagmus are cerebellar impairments, head trauma, toxic-metabolic insults, and congenital factors.

Down-beating nystagmus can also be caused by drug intoxication (e.g., lithium and antiepileptic medications).

Up-Beating Nystagmus

Up-beating nystagmus that is central in origin is characterized by a nystagmus with a fast phase beating upward when the patient's eyes are in the primary position (Figure 5–28) (Bojrab & McFeely, 2001). Impairments that cause this form of nystagmus are not as localized as those that cause down-beating nystagmus; however, it has been reported primarily in patients with impairments in the dorsal paramedian caudal medulla and pontine and midbrain lesions (Leigh & Zee, 2006). One important clinical note is that the examiner should differentiate a centrally generated up-beating nystagmus from posterior canal BPPV (benign paroxysmal positional vertigo, transient up-beating nystagmus with changes in head position). Up-beating nystagmus that is present in primary position often follows Alexander's law (largest intensity during upward gaze). Up-beating nystagmus does not typically increase with lateral gaze as does down-beating nystagmus, although when the patient tilts their head upward, the nystagmus may reverse (Leigh & Zee, 2006). As with down-beating nystagmus, up-beating nystagmus of central origin is not fully suppressed by visual fixation and patients often complain of impaired gait, unsteadiness, and oscillopsia (Leigh & Zee,

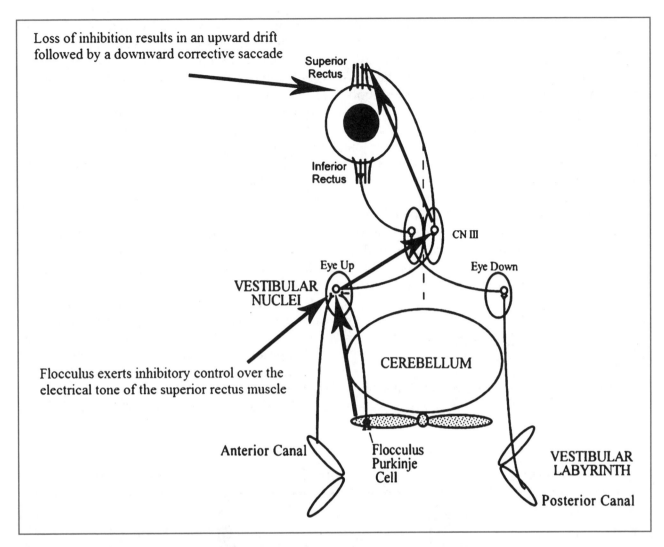

Loss of inhibition results in an upward drift
followed by a downward corrective saccade

Flocculus exerts inhibitory control over the
electrical tone of the superior rectus muscle

FIGURE 5–27. A hypothetical schematic by Ito et al. (1977) illustrates the origin of down-beating nystagmus. The flocculus of the cerebellum inhibits the anterior semicircular canal but not the posterior projections. If inhibition is impaired, the eyes drift upward. Down-beating nystagmus is composed of the slow drift of the eye upward and the corrective saccade downward. (From Leigh & Zee, 2006)

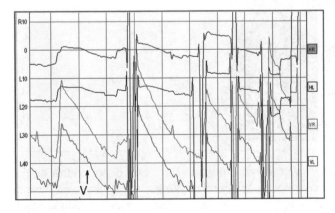

FIGURE 5–28. Up-beating nystagmus at center gaze is shown.

2006). Up-beating nystagmus is commonly associated with lesions of the medulla, midbrain, and cerebellum (Leigh & Zee, 2006). Other causes of up-beating nystagmus are stroke, multiple sclerosis, congenital factors, and tumors. It can also be caused by tobacco abuse and middle ear disease, and it must be differentiated from posterior semicircular canal BPPV.

Brun's Nystagmus

Brun's nystagmus is a variant of nystagmus that is characterized by a combination of both central GEN and peripheral vestibular nystagmus (Bruns,

1908; Croxson et al., 1988). Brun's nystagmus is typically observed in patients suffering from large cerebellopontine-angle tumors (e.g., commonly vestibular schwannomas or acoustic neuromas) that are large enough to compress both the ipsilateral eighth cranial nerve and the cerebellar flocculus. The result is a spontaneous peripheral vestibular nystagmus with a fast phase beating toward the contralesional ear while the impairment in the cerebellar flocculus generates a GEN "beating" toward the ipsilesional gaze direction (Figure 5–29). The presence of Brun's nystagmus typically indicates that the patient has a large tumor (>3.5 cm) (Lloyd et al., 2009; Nedzelski, 1983; Baloh, Konrad, Dirks, & Honrubia, 1976; Okada, Takahashi, Saito, & Kanzaki, 1991).

Nystagmus of Peripheral Origin (Vestibulopathy)

Nystagmus of peripheral origin (vestibular labyrinth or nerve) that changes intensity with gaze is most commonly generated by an uncompensated asymmetry in neural input from the two labyrinths (see Chapter 3 for a more complete review). When interpreting the spontaneous nystagmus test it is important that the clinician have laboratory-specific normative data to compare with the patient findings. This prevents overinterpretation and unnecessary referrals for additional studies. K. Barin (personal communication) has reported that in his laboratory, spontaneous horizontal nystagmus with vision denied must be greater than 6° per second for ENG and 4° per second for VNG to be considered abnormal. Additionally, vertical nystagmus must exceed 7° per second with vision denied when using VNG. In cases where patients are seen acutely following an attack of peripheral vertigo, this form of nystagmus can be observed during the gaze test. In patients suffering from peripheral impairments, spontaneous nystagmus that is present with fixation is typically observed only acutely. Peripherally generated nystagmus is characterized by a mixed horizontal and torsional nystagmus with the fast phase directed

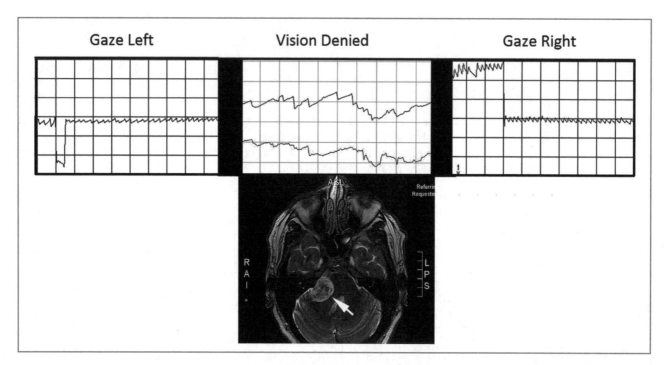

FIGURE 5–29. Brun's nystagmus. The patient presented with a 3-cm mass in right cerebellopontine angle that extended into the internal auditory canal. Note the spontaneous peripheral vestibular nystagmus with vision denied. With lateral gaze, characteristics of the nystagmus change (i.e., low-amplitude high-frequency bidirectional nystagmus).

away from the ipsilesional ear. The intensity of the nystagmus increases when the eyes are deviated in the direction of the fast phase (Alexander's law). Alexander's law refers to peripherally generated nystagmus that is observed with the eyes open. It is qualified by degrees of severity. With the first degree, nystagmus is observed only during lateral gaze in the direction of the quick phase (Figure 5–30). With the second degree, nystagmus is present in the primary position with the lateral gaze in the direction of the quick phases (Figure 5–31). With the third degree, nystagmus is present in the primary gaze with the lateral gaze in both directions (Figure 5–32). A classic sign that the observed nystagmus is peripheral in origin is that it reduces in intensity with visual fixation and increases in intensity when vision is denied. Peripherally generated nystagmus has a linear slow component and is direction fixed. (For a complete discussion of peripherally generated vestibular nystagmus see Chapter 2.)

SMOOTH PURSUIT TRACKING TEST

The testing of the functional eye class smooth pursuit is accomplished by recording the patient's eye movements while they track a target moving in

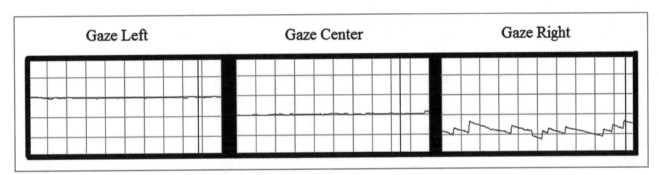

FIGURE 5–30. First-degree direction-fixed spontaneous vestibular nystagmus in the gaze positions. Note that the nystagmus is present only during right gaze (i.e., the direction of the fast phase). This case illustrates a 47-year-old man with a history of a left temporal bone fracture incurred 3 days before the recordings were taken. The patient reports both continuous disequilibrium and positional vertigo.

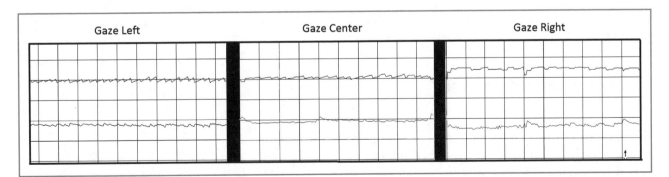

FIGURE 5–31. Second-degree left-beating direction-fixed spontaneous vestibular nystagmus. Note that the nystagmus is present in center and left gaze but not when gaze is directed to the right. This case illustrates a 51-year-old man with a history of vertiginous episodes that occur approximately three times per week and last 30–40 min. The vertigo is accompanied by aural fullness and tinnitus in the right ear. The patient carries a provisional diagnosis of Ménière disease.

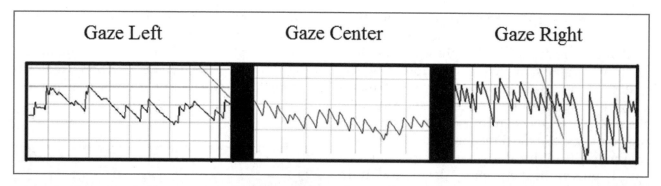

FIGURE 5–32. Third-degree right-beating direction-fixed spontaneous vestibular nystagmus. Note that the nystagmus is present in center, left, and right gaze. This case illustrates a 49-year-old man with a history of vertigo that has been ongoing for the past 5 years. The attacks of vertigo are followed by periods where the patient is asymptomatic. The patient's last attack was 1 day before the recordings were obtained.

a sinusoidal trajectory in the horizontal plane. Today's targets are typically displayed on a light bar or projected onto a wall in front of the patient.

Assessment of Smooth Pursuit

In order to perform smooth pursuit testing, the patient should be instructed to maintain the head in the midline position and follow the target with their eyes. It is important to communicate to the patient that they should keep their attention directed toward the stimulus for the duration of the test. The visual stimulus should make an excursion of 30° to the right and 30° to the left at a range of frequencies (0.2–0.8 Hz). Smooth pursuit performance degrades with age; thus, when testing, age-corrected normative data should be employed. When an abnormality (e.g., saccadic pursuit) is observed, the test should be repeated.

Interpretation and Analysis

The three primary parameters that are used for the clinical analysis of pursuit are how close the eye movement is to the movement of the target, the difference in percent between the left eye and right eye, and whether the eye is leading or lagging the target. When interpreting the smooth pursuit test, the recordings should be examined for the presence of any GEN, spontaneous vestibular nystagmus, or saccadic intrusions. The sec-

tions below provide the primary parameters that are used for the analysis of smooth pursuit.

Velocity Gain

Velocity gain is the relationship between the velocity of the eye and the velocity of the target at a given time. Specifically, velocity gain describes how closely the output signal (eye) matches the input signal (target) at a certain point in time. If the eye velocity (in degrees per second) is equal to the target velocity (in degrees per second) at the time of measurement, the gain is 1. If the eye falls behind the target, when the measurement is made the target (input) velocity will be greater than the eye (output) velocity and the value will be less than 1. As is seen in Figure 5–33, abnormal gain is in the lower region (<1). This is typically considered to be a sign of central impairment. The abnormal region represented by the shaded area and displays two standard deviations from mean age-corrected normative data.

The following equation defines velocity gain:

$$\text{Velocity gain} = \frac{\text{Peak eye velocity (degrees/second)}}{\text{Peak target velocity (degrees/second)}}$$

Asymmetry

Asymmetry reflects the difference in velocity gain (described above) between rightward eye move-

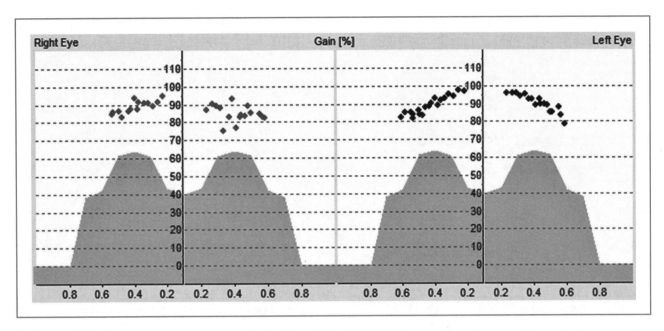

FIGURE 5–33. A image of how pursuit velocity gain is plotted (Interacoustics, Assens, Denmark).

ments and leftward eye movements. This can often be abnormal in cases where a patient is generating spontaneous nystagmus. For example, if the patient has right-beating spontaneous nystagmus, the patient typically manifests abnormally reduced velocity gain on the right.

Phase Angle

Phase angle refers to the measurement of how much the eye is leading or lagging the visual target. The value is calculated in degrees and provides a measure of how in phase the eyes are with the target (e.g., an eye movement that is 180° out of phase with the target suggests that the eye is moving in the opposite direction (Figure 5–34). When the patient's eyes are continually ahead of the target, they should be reinstructed.

Pursuit Abnormalities

Patients with impairments affecting the pursuit system most commonly replace the smooth pursuit of the target with a series of saccadic eye movements. Saccadic pursuit occurs when the patient's eyes lag behind the target and the oculo-

motor system must generate a saccadic eye movement to reacquire it. This series of events results in a stepped response rather than the smooth sinusoidal response that is observed in normal patients. Saccadic pursuit is typically analyzed as reduced gain (eye velocity divided by target velocity) and is often referred to in the literature as "cogwheeling." Saccadic pursuit is also occasionally observed in normal patients. Specifically, if the clinician notices that the patient's eyes are being taken off the target and jumping ahead, it may indicate a lack of concentration or alertness and reinstruction regarding the task should be administered. The pursuit pathway sends projections to numerous regions of the brain and brainstem and thus has limited clinical utility for localizing the site of lesion. For example, abnormal pursuit is observed in patients with impairments affecting the vestibular nuclei, cerebellum, dorsolateral pontine nuclei, striate cortex, middle temporal areas of the cortex, and the frontal eye fields (Kandel, Schwartz, & Jessell, 2000); however, abnormal pursuit can also be the result of medications, inattention, and cooperation. When a pursuit impairment is confirmed, Leigh and Zee (2006) report that it is typically more severe when the lower-level generators are involved (i.e., brainstem).

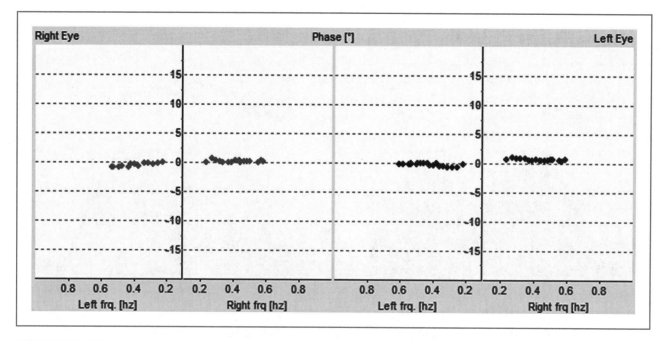

FIGURE 5–34. A image of how pursuit asymmetry is plotted (Interacoustics, Assens, Denmark).

Bilaterally Saccadic Pursuit

Overall, bilaterally reduced smooth pursuit is of little or no diagnostic utility. Bilaterally low-gain pursuit responses are found in patients with disorders affecting the visual system as well as the central and peripheral vestibular systems. For this reason, the examiner should exercise caution when attempting to diagnose impairments based on findings from pursuit testing alone. Hain (1992) has suggested categorizing bilaterally reduced pursuit responses into three types. First, pursuit is considered normal if the gain parameter is greater than 0.8 Hz. Second, pursuit gains of greater than 0.2, but less than 0.8, are considered to be in a "gray zone." In these cases interpretation should include findings from other tests before making a decision regarding whether the examination is normal or abnormal. Finally, patients with a gain of less than 0.2 are considered to have significant pursuit abnormalities (Hain, 1992). Impairments can range from the level of the cortex to the cerebellum and brainstem (a very diffuse circuit making localization of the impairment difficult). Bilaterally saccadic pursuit can be caused by brainstem disease, cerebellar impairments, and cerebral hemisphere impairments. When bilater-

ally saccadic pursuit tracing are encountered, caution should be exercised to rule out medication, inattention, fatigue, inattentive head movement, and congenital nystagmus.

Figure 5–35 shows a pursuit recording of a patient with multiple sclerosis in the brainstem and cerebellum. There is a significant degree of saccade pursuit bilaterally.

Unilaterally Saccadic Pursuit

When a patient generates pursuit that is asymmetric, the clinician must determine if the origin is central or peripheral. When spontaneous nystagmus originating from an acute peripheral vestibular disorder is present, the oculomotor system is generating a sawtooth waveform (slow and fast phase). In other words, the asymmetry in tonic neural activity between the two vestibular systems activates the VOR and the eyes are driven slowly toward the impaired ear until they reach a point in the orbit and are quickly reset in the direction of the intact ear. Patients with spontaneous vestibular nystagmus often produce unilaterally impaired tracking waveforms (asymmetric low gain) because the oculomotor system is unable

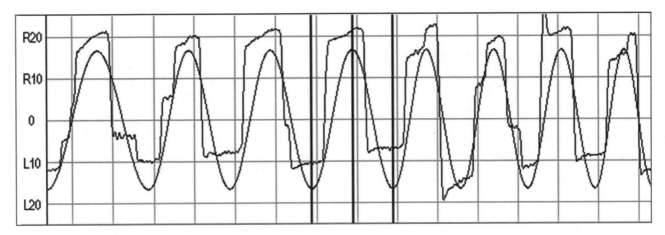

FIGURE 5–35. A recording of bilaterally saccadic pursuit is shown.

to integrate the fast phase of the aberrant spontaneous nystagmus and the smooth pursuit movement generated by the tracking system. When the patient is instructed to follow the smooth pursuit target in the direction of the slow phase of the nystagmus, the gain (eye movement/target movement) is essentially equivalent; however, when the patient is requested to pursue targets in the direction of the spontaneous nystagmus fast phase, the resulting pursuit waveform will either be low in amplitude (i.e., low pursuit gain) or absent entirely (Figure 5–36). In central cases, the pursuit system cannot accurately compute the target velocity resulting in the use of saccades to track the target (Heide et al., 1996). Central causes of unilaterally saccadic pursuit include impairments in the cortex (parietal and frontal lobe), thalamus, midbrain, cerebellum, and dorsolateral pontine nuclei. Cortical impairments typically degrade smooth pursuit performance in the direction ipsilateral to the impairment (Heide et al., 1996).

OPTOKINETIC TEST

The optokinetic test (OKN) is accomplished by having a patient watch a series of stimuli moving horizontally across their visual field while recording their eye movements. The primary purpose of the OKN system is to stabilize objects of interest when the head is moving (originally referred to as "railway" nystagmus). In this regard, in order to generate a "true" OKN nystagmus the observer's visual field should be 90% or more filled with stimuli. Using a full-field visual stimulus will evoke circular-vection (i.e., the subjective perception of circular motion) (Leigh & Zee, 2006). Full-field stimulation of the visual field cannot, in most instances, be achieved using the light bars that come with many commercially available ENG/VNG systems. OKN responses generated using stimuli delivered via a light bar are volitional and are activating primarily the pursuit system. These responses are referred to as "look" OKN responses (Shepard & Schubert, 2008). In contrast, the true reflexive, brainstem-mediated OKN response generated using full-field visual stimulation is known as "stare" OKN. In order to generate "stare" OKN responses most systems employ a projector system or present the stimuli inside a rotational chair enclosure (Figure 5–37). OKN stimuli consist of high contrast patterns that consist of stripes or circles. Recently, stimuli employing images (e.g., trains or playground scenes) have been employed for use with children and have been shown to produce OKN responses equivalent to conventional stimuli (D. L. McCaslin, C. Bahner, and B. Wengar, unpublished findings). The instructions provided to the patient are important in obtaining robust OKN responses. Patients who choose to "look through" the OKN pattern can significantly reduce the gain. Patients should be instructed to keep their head very still and simply look at the pattern as it passes by. Because of the diffuse projections,

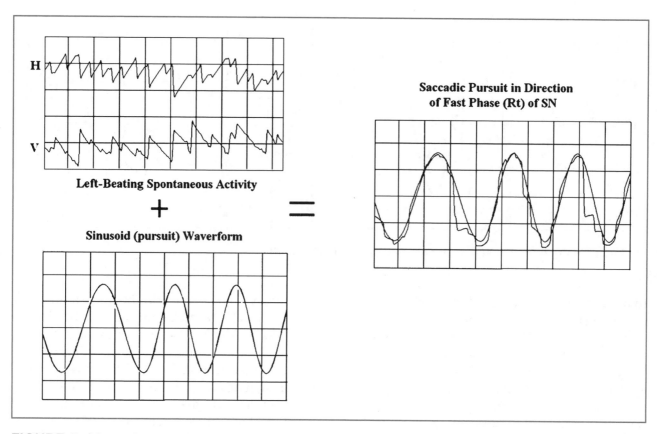

FIGURE 5–36. The effect that spontaneous vestibular nystagmus has on the pursuit test. Note that the eye movement system cannot integrate both a smooth and a fast eye movement. **SN** Spontaneous nystagmus; **H** horizontal; **V** vertical. (From McCaslin & Jacobson, 2009)

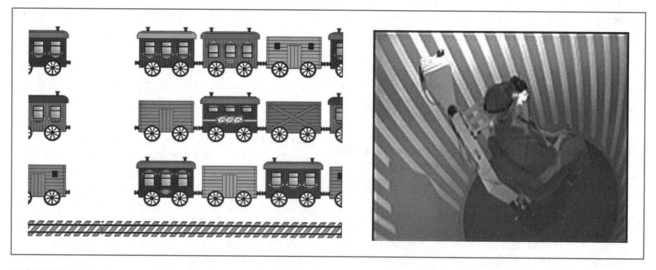

FIGURE 5–37. A. An example of the type of stimuli that can be employed using projectors for the generation of optokinetic stimuli. **B.** An example of a patient in the rotary chair being subjected to a full-field optokinetic stimulus.

OKN ("stare") testing, like pursuit, is of limited diagnostic utility; however, unlike the pursuit system, the response is reflexive and is not as heavily influenced by inattention or medication. The two primary paradigms for evaluating the OKN system are fixed and sinusoidal.

The section below outlines the technique for the fixed paradigm. (Readers are referred to Shepard and Schubert [2008] for a more comprehensive discussion regarding the assessment of OKN [e.g., sinusoidal and optokinetic after-nystagmus paradigms].)

Assessment of the Optokinetic System

In order to perform optokinetic testing, the patient should be instructed to maintain the head in the midline position and look *straight ahead* at the pattern as it moves across the screen or wall. Furthermore, the patient should be asked to "look" and focus on the stimuli as they pass by, and not to ignore them. It is important to communicate to the patient that they should be careful not to select one stimulus and follow it as that will invoke the smooth pursuit system. The visual stimulus should consist of a full-field stimulus moving at a constant velocity at 20° per second and 35–40° per second in both directions. Recordings should be taken for a minimum of 30 s. When an abnormality (e.g., reduced gain) is observed the test should be repeated.

Interpretation and Analysis

As with pursuit testing, the primary parameter that is evaluated during the assessment of OKN is velocity gain. A gain measure is calculated for targets moving to the right and left and then compared using an asymmetry formula. There are two primary OKN abnormalities when the fixed paradigm is employed. First, gain can be bilaterally reduced. Secondly, gain can demonstrate a significant asymmetry (e.g., the response to the rightward-moving field is smaller than the response to the leftward-moving field. The calculated asymmetry should not exceed 25% (Shepard & Schubert, 2008). It is noteworthy that each clinician should have norma-

tive data, as the calculations and analysis methods used to calculate these values are often proprietary and vary between manufacturers.

Velocity Gain

Velocity gain is the relationship between the velocity of the eye and the velocity of the OKN stimulus. Specifically, velocity gain describes how closely the slow phase of the nystagmus (eye) matches the velocity of the optokinetic field.

The following equation defines OKN velocity gain:

$$\text{OKN velocity gain} = \frac{\text{Peak eye velocity (degrees/second)}}{\text{Peak target velocity (degrees/second)}}$$

Asymmetry

Asymmetry reflects the difference in velocity gain (described above) between rightward and leftward eye movements. This can often be abnormal in cases where a patient is generating spontaneous nystagmus. For example, if the patient has right-beating spontaneous nystagmus, the patient typically manifests abnormally reduced velocity gain on the right.

Optokinetic Abnormalities

An abnormality in the OKN system has been reported to occur when the gain for a 60° per second stimulus is less than 0.56 (Baloh & Furman, 1989). It is important to note that normal OKN gain is not the same for all target velocities. Specifically, OKN gain decreases as the speed of the targets is increased.

Bilaterally Reduced Optokinetic Responses

Symmetrically reduced optokinetic responses can occur for a number of reasons. First, the presence of a disorder in the pursuit system manifests bilaterally reduced gain. When performing the pursuit task, the fovea must be kept directly on the target;

however, the OKN response is evoked by both central (foveal) and peripheral (extrafoveal) vision and is the reason that a full-field stimulus is used. In patients with impairments in central vision, the examiner commonly observes reduced OKN gain at the beginning of the test and increasing OKN as the test progresses (Baloh, Yee, & Honrubia, 1980). In patients with impairments in their peripheral vision, but have normal central vision, this increase in gain is not observed. Another abnormality that contributes to symmetrically reduced OKN gain is a saccade impairment. Patients with disease in the brainstem where the pulse neurons for the generation of saccades are located are unable to generate the fast phase that is required to reset the eye during the OKN response. This inability of the patient to quickly bring the eye back to center results in the gain of the OKN response being significantly reduced (Figure 5–38). This inability to generate saccades is often observed during caloric and rotational testing and can be mistaken for a weakness in the bilateral peripheral vestibular system. Other sources of bilaterally reduced optokinetic responses include impairments in the cortex to the cerebellum. Whenever bilaterally reduced OKN is observed caution should be exercised to rule out

medication, visual impairments, inattention, and inattentive head movement.

Unilaterally Reduced Optokinetic Responses

The finding of a significant asymmetry during optokinetic testing can suggest either a central nervous system impairment or the presence of spontaneous vestibular nystagmus. As explained in the previous section detailing abnormalities in the pursuit system, the oculomotor system has difficulty integrating the fast phase of the spontaneous nystagmus and the slow movement of the target (Figure 5–39). This can lead to asymmetrically reduced OKN gain when the direction of the OKN stimulus beats in the opposite direction of the fast phase of the spontaneous nystagmus; however, it is noteworthy that asymmetric pursuit can be observed in patients with impairments in the temporal lobes, unilateral parieto-occipital disorders, and the brainstem. If a central cause is suspected, other tests of oculomotor function (e.g., gaze and saccades) should be carefully inspected and the presence of any spontaneous nystagmus should be ruled out.

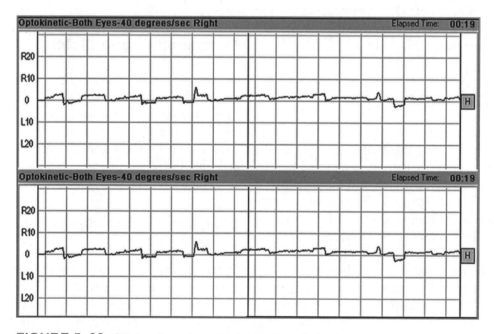

FIGURE 5–38. Bilaterally reduced optokinetic gain is shown.

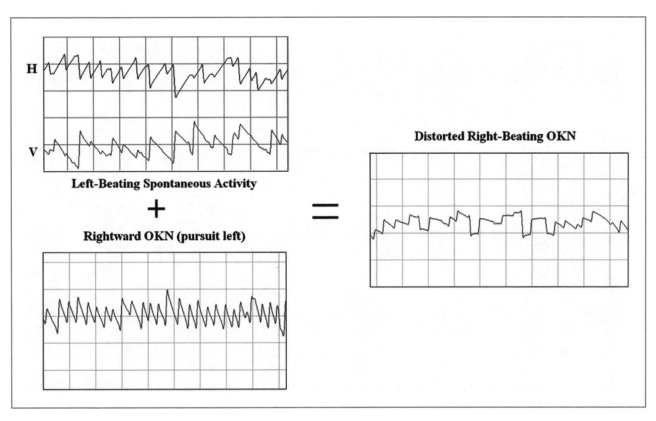

FIGURE 5–39. The effect that spontaneous vestibular nystagmus has on "look" optokinetic tests. Note that the eye movement system cannot integrate both a smooth and a fast eye movement. **OKN** Optokinetic nystagmus; **H** horizontal; **V** vertical. (From McCaslin & Jacobson, 2009)

‖‖‖ 6 ‖‖‖

Positional and Positioning Testing

Introduction

The purpose of positional testing is twofold. First, the test is performed to document the patient's complaint of position-induced vertigo and/or dizziness. The second reason is to record the effect that gravity, and static body positions, has on the tonic afferent neural output originating from the peripheral vestibular system. Patients with both peripheral and central vestibular system impairments can generate position-induced nystagmus.

Background

Static positioning testing involves recording a patient's eye movements with the head placed in a sequence of different positions. Each position changes the orientation of the head with respect to the earth gravitational vector and can subsequently modulate the baseline "neural tone" in the vestibular system (Coats, 1993); thus, the purpose of this test is to document (through eye recordings) the presence or modulation of position-induced nystagmus, and, to the extent possible, determine whether the nystagmus is originating from the peripheral vestibular sys-

tem or the central vestibular system (Brandt, 1990; Baloh & Honrubia, 2001; Leigh & Zee, 2006). A comprehensive list of the causes of nystagmus associated with changes in head position is provided in Table 6–1. It is noteworthy that not all positional nystagmus is of clinical significance. There continues to be disagreement in the literature as to whether there is a high percentage of the normal population that presents with positional nystagmus (Barber & Wright, 1973; Coats, 1993; McAuley, Dickman, Mustain, & Anand, 1996). For example, in a landmark study examining positional nystagmus in normal subjects, Barber and Wright (1973) reported that 82% of their randomly selected sample of 112 participants had measureable positional nystagmus. This finding that positional nystagmus is observed in the majority of normal subjects has been supported by others (McAuley et al., 1996). In contrast to these findings, Van der Stappen et al. (2000) and Hajioff, Barr-Hamilton, College, Lewis, and Wilson (2000) reported positional nystagmus in their control sample of 7.5 and 27%, respectively. This failure to find consensus is related to investigators using a multitude of different positions and analysis techniques. For these reasons the observation of nystagmus or vertigo induced by static position testing is, in most instances, of minor diagnostic utility. The one factor that does discriminate between central and peripheral positional nystagmus is fixation ability. Positional nystagmus due

Table 6–1. Nystagmus and Vertigo Associated with Changes in Head Position

Vertigo and/or Nystagmus Associated with Head Motion or Changes in Head Position Relative to the Gravitational Vector
Central vestibular (pontomedullary brainstem of vestibulocerebellum)
Positional down-beating nystagmus
Down-beating nystagmus/vertigo
Up-beating nystagmus/vertigo
Central positional nystagmus without major vertigo
Central positional vertigo with nystagmus
Basilar insufficiency
Vestibular nerve
Neurovascular compression ("disabling positional vertigo")
Peripheral labyrinth
Benign paroxysmal positional vertigo
Cupula/endolymph gravity differential (buoyancy mechanism)
Positional alcohol vertigo/nystagmus
Positional "heavy water" nystagmus
Positional glycerol nystagmus
Positional nystagmus with macroglobulinemia
Perilymph fistula
Ménière disease
Vestibular atelectasia
Physiologic "head-extension vertigo" or "bending-over vertigo"
Vestibular head-motion intolerance (oscillopsia and unsteadiness of gait)
Bilateral vestibulopathy
Oculomotor disorders (defective vestibulo-ocular reflex)
Neurovascular cross-compression ("vestibular paroxysmia")
Vestibulocerebellar ataxia
Perilymphatic fistula
Post-traumatic otolith vertigo
Vestibulocerebellar intoxication (e.g., alcohol, phenytoin)

Source: From Brandt, 1993

to impairment in the peripheral vestibular system can almost always be significantly attenuated with visual fixation. For this reason static positioning testing is initially performed without fixation (vision denied). If nystagmus is observed during a position with vision denied (no fixation), the test should be repeated with fixation. The patient should be given mental alerting tasks during the test.

Technique

The technique for static positional testing (Figure 6–1) is as follows:

1. Perform the search for spontaneous nystagmus (sitting) and positioning testing before assessing static positional testing.

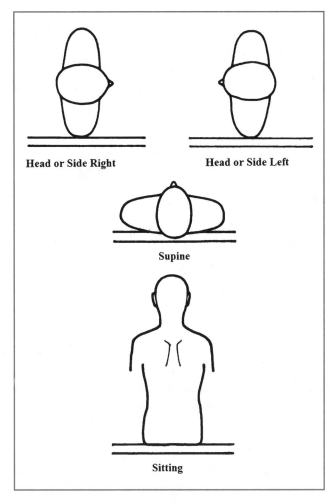

FIGURE 6–1. The primary positions used during the static position test. (From Brandt, 1993)

2. Prepare to provide a mental-alerting task for the patient for each position. The patient should be wearing videonystagmography goggles or Frenzel's glasses with eyes open.

3. Lay the patient in the recumbent position (supine) with vision denied for 30 s.

   a. If nystagmus is present following 30 s of recording, maintain the patient in this position for 2 min (allows differentiation between positional nystagmus and benign paroxysmal positional vertigo).

   b. If the nystagmus continues at a constant intensity, instruct the patient to fixate on a target.

   c. Record the effect of fixation on the nystagmus (i.e., determine if fixation significantly reduces the observed nystagmus).

4. Repeat the sequence in step 3 for head right or body right (body right can be used if patient presents with cervical spondylosis, osteoarthritis, did not have any measurable nystagmus during spontaneous testing, or has a restricted cervical range of motion).

5. Repeat the sequence in step 3 for head left or body left.

6. Repeat the sequence in step 3 with the patient supine with neck flexion at 30°.

Interpretation

When interpreting positional nystagmus it is important that the findings be correlated with the quantitative vestibular function test results as well as the case history. In order to appropriately determine if static positional nystagmus is pathologic (i.e., peripheral or central), the examiner should be able to answer four primary questions. First, what is the peak amplitude of the observed nystagmus (e.g., average of three beats)? When recording using VNG, if the slow-phase velocity of any observed horizontal nystagmus is greater than 4° per second (7° per second for vertical nystagmus) in any of the static positions, then further analysis should be undertaken (Barin, 2008b). Second, how long does the response last (intermittent or persistent)? This question serves to determine if the nystagmus observed is a form of benign paroxysmal positioning vertigo (BPPV) or if it is positional nystagmus generated by an asymmetry in the vestibulo-ocular reflex (VOR) pathway. Third, is the nystagmus direction fixed or direction-changing in one or more head positions? The presence of a positional nystagmus that changes direction in a single head position is diagnostic for intracranial disease, usually affecting the cerebellar system (i.e., cerebellum and pons). When horizontal nystagmus is not observed during either the sitting or supine positions but is measurable during the head left or head right position, the examiner should consider the effect of neck rotation. The effect of neck rotation can be ruled out by retesting the patient in the body left and body right positions. If there is no measurable nystagmus during the body right or body left position, the observed nystagmus is most likely due to neck torsion (e.g., "cerviogenic dizziness/

nystagmus"). Finally, what is the effect of fixation on the intensity of the positional nystagmus? A positional nystagmus that cannot be attenuated with visual fixation implicates abnormal function of the reciprocal connections between the midline cerebellar structures and pons. In many instances, a significant horizontal positional nystagmus that can be attenuated with visual fixation is found in the presence of a unilateral peripheral vestibular system impairment. Tables 6–2 and 6–3 present

Table 6–2. Duration of Observed Nystagmus

Finding	Significance/Comments
Intermittent nystagmus	Rule out BPPV and patient lack of alertness
Persistent nystagmus	Significant if peak SPV is >6° per second for ENG (no fixation)
	Significant if peak SPV is >4° per second for VNG (no fixation) (Barin, 2008b)
	Significant if nystagmus of any intensity does not diminish with fixation

BPPV benign paroxysmal positioning vertigo; *SPV* slow-phase velocity

Table 6–3. Characteristics of the Nystagmus and the Effect of Fixation

Finding	Fixation	No Fixation	Significance/Comments
Direction-fixed horizontal nystagmus	Decreases significantly (50%) or is abolished	Enhances	Peripheral (vestibular nystagmus)
Direction-fixed horizontal nystagmus	Decreases significantly (50%) or is abolished	Present	Normal
Vertical nystagmus	No decrease	Present	Central abnormality (up-beating or down-beating) (Baloh & Honrubia, 1990; Pierrot-Deseilligny & Milea, 2005).
Vertical nystagmus <7° per second (VNG)	Decreases significantly (50%) or is abolished	Present	Normal (Barin, 2008b)
Direction-changing horizontal nystagmus (apogeotropic)	Decreases significantly (50%)	Present	Right oblique positional alcohol nystagmus and HSC BPPV
Direction-changing horizontal nystagmus (geotropic)	Decreases significantly (50%)	Present	Right oblique positional alcohol nystagmus and HSC BPPV
Direction-fixed horizontal nystagmus	No decrease in intensity	No increase in intensity	Suggests central impairment
Direction-changing horizontal nystagmus in a single head position	Present	Present	Rule out periodic alternating nystagmus; central finding
Direction-changing horizontal nystagmus in a single head position	Abolished	Present	Central finding

HSC horizontal semicircular canal; *BPPV* benign paroxysmal positioning vertigo

a summary of potential findings for each of the questions and their significance.

Two flow charts recently reported by Barin (2008b) have summarized the interpretation of both horizontal (Figure 6–2) and vertical nystagmus (Figure 6–3) during the static positional test. These decision pathways can be used as a simple and effective way to guide the clinician through the process of interpreting whether observed positional nystagmus is of clinical significance.

Positional Alcohol Nystagmus

As discussed in the previous section, nystagmus resulting from impairment in the peripheral ves-

tibular system is typically direction fixed; however, one type of nystagmus that is peripheral in origin and changes direction with different head positions is positional alcohol nystagmus (PAN). Caution should be exercised when using the acronym PAN so that positional alcohol nystagmus is not confused with periodic alternating nystagmus. Alcohol consumed by a patient initially enters the bloodstream and then the cupula and endolymph. The mechanism behind PAN involves the ingested alcohol reaching the cupula before it reaches the endolymph. Because the density of alcohol is lighter than surrounding endolymph, the cupula becomes lighter and will float (like a bobber). This action will produce nystagmus during positional testing has been termed PAN I. The main

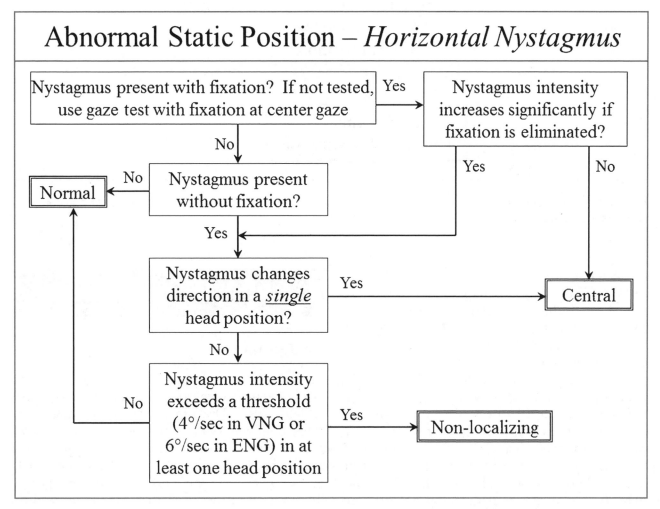

FIGURE 6–2. Algorithm for the interpretation of horizontal nystagmus observed during the static position test. (Courtesy of Kamran Barin)

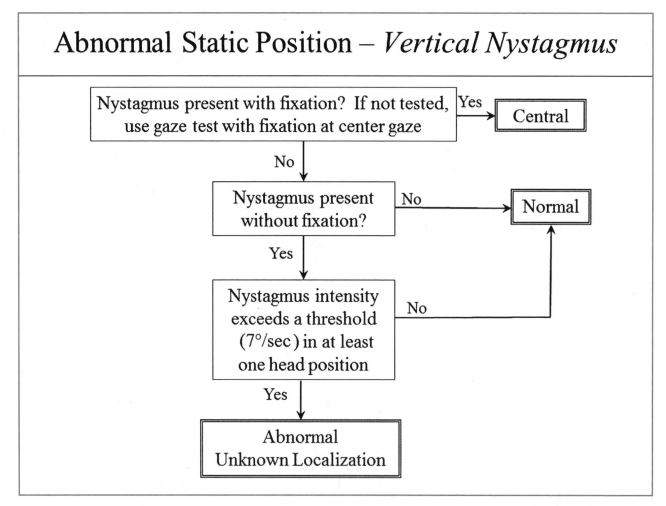

FIGURE 6–3. Algorithm for the interpretation of vertical nystagmus observed during the static position test. (Courtesy of Kamran Barin)

characteristic of PAN I (i.e., resorption phase of PAN) is direction-changing *geotropic* nystagmus with head right or left (Figure 6–4A). Alternatively, alcohol is absorbed by the body earlier in the cupula than in the endolymph causing the cupula to sink (like a sinker) and has been referred to as PAN II. PAN II (i.e., reduction phase of PAN) generates an apogeotropic nystagmus during positional testing (Figure 6–4B). Approximately 2–5 hours following the ingestion of a significant amount of alcohol, there will be a "window" between PAN I and PAN II where there is no observable positional nystagmus. This "intermediate period" exists when alcohol has diffused into both the cupula and the endolymph and the specific gravity becomes equal again.

POSITIONING TESTING

Background

Benign paroxysmal positioning vertigo (BPPV) is one of the most common forms of vertigo (Hotson & Baloh, 1998; Drachman 1998; Furman & Cass, 1999; Bhattacharyya et al., 2008). Barany (1907) provided the initial description of this type of dizziness that is characterized by intense, but brief, vertigo and nystagmus provoked by changes in the position of the head. BPPV is the term most commonly used to describe the disorder with this specific set of symptoms. "Benign" refers to

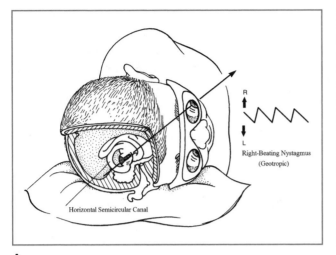

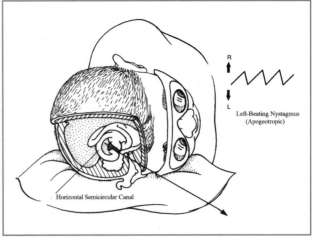

A   **B**

FIGURE 6–4. **A** and **B.** Eye movements and physiologic mechanism of positional alcohol nystagmus (PAN). **A.** PAN I generates geotropic nystagmus. **B.** PANII generates apogeotropic nystagmus. (Courtesy of Daniel Pender, adapted from Pender, 1992)

the fact that the disorder is peripheral and can often be successfully treated. The word "paroxysmal" means a brief, violent outburst. "Positioning" refers to the fact that in order to provoke the symptoms, the head (and consequently the semicircular canals) must be moved into certain positions. Finally, "vertigo" implies that the patient perceives his or her surroundings to be moving when he or she is not moving. During the case history, patients with BPPV often report that the dizziness occurs when they roll over in bed, look up, or bend over. In this vein, Whitney, Marchetti, and Morris (2005) reported that five items on the Dizziness Handicap Inventory (DHI) can help the clinician in the identification of patients with BPPV. The five items include the following:

1. Does looking up increase your problem?
2. Because of your problem, do you have difficulty getting into or out of bed?
3. Do quick movements of your head increase your problem?
4. Does turning over in bed increase your problem?
5. Does bending over increase your problem?

Patients with BPPV had significantly higher mean scores than those who did not have BPPV. Spe-

cifically, the authors reported that scores on the five-item abbreviated BPPV DHI were predictive of patients with BPPV (Whitney et al., 2005).

The confirmation of BPPV is based on a set of maneuvers designed to induce the nystagmus and vertigo in each of the canals. The first maneuver described to specifically provoke BPPV was reported by Margaret Dix and Charles Hallpike in 1952 using their sample of 100 patients at Queen Square Hospital (Dix & Hallpike, 1952). In this maneuver, the patient sits on the exam table with the head turned 45° toward the side being tested and then is brought to the supine position with the head extended off the edge of the table. The authors reported a torsional vertical nystagmus beating toward the dependent ear that was brief in duration and reversed direction upon having the patient sit up. This maneuver, known as the Dix-Hallpike maneuver, continues to be part of the assessment of the dizziness patient.

Epidemiology

Several groups of investigators have reported on the incidence (the risk of developing a condition within a specified period of time) and prevalence (the total number of cases of the condition in the population at a given time) of BPPV in the general population. Approximately 6 million people per year enter the United States health care system with complaints of dizziness. According to Bhattacharyya et al. (2008), 17–42% of these patients are diagnosed with BPPV. Accordingly, the prevalence of BPPV ranges from 10.7 to 64 per 100,000 in the general population with a lifetime prevalence of 2.5% (Bhattacharyya et al., 2008). Findings are similar in other countries as well. For instance, Mizukoshi et al. (1988) described the incidence of BPPV in Japan to be 10.7–17.3 per 100,000. von Brevern et al. (2007) conducted a cross-sectional study of the general population in Europe and reported a lifetime prevalence of 2.4%. Age is also a significant factor to be considered when reporting on the incidence and prevalence of BPPV. Froehling et al. (1991) presented data from a retrospective review of medical records in health care systems in the United States of patients presenting with BPPV. The authors reported that the patients seeking medical attention for BPPV increased by 38% with each decade of life (mean age 51 years). There are other studies supporting the fact that BPPV is more prevalent in the elderly (von Brevern et al., 2007; Baloh, Honrubia, & Jacobson, 1987). Hilton and Pinder (2004) reported that the peak incidence of BPPV occurs between 50 and 70 years. In elderly patients BPPV can have serious consequences. In a cross-sectional investigation by Oghalai, Manolidis, Barth, Stewart, and Jenkins (2000), elderly patients presenting with BPPV were shown to limit their activity level and have a greater incidence of falls. Furthermore, 9% of the participants in their study had unrecognized BPPV (Oghalai et al., 2000). Originally, the term "benign" in BPPV was included because this type of vertigo is peripheral and can be managed in most instances; however, those who experience it would agree that, when triggered, the sensation of BPPV is anything but "benign." Also, because elderly persons with BPPV are at a greater risk of falling, the term "benign" is a misnomer. BPPV does occasionally occur in younger patients who have suffered a head trauma, present with migraine, or have had a procedure that keeps them bedridden for an extended period of time.

The majority of patients with positioning vertigo present with BPPV that affects either the posterior (PSC-BPPV) or the horizontal semicircular canal (HSC-BPPV). PSC-BPPV has been reported to make up 85–90% of all BPPV cases (Parnes, Agrawal, & Atlas, 2003). HSC-BPPV accounts for 5–15% of cases of BPPV (Cakir et al., 2006; Parnes et al., 2003). The incidence of BPPV among the three semicircular canals (SCCs), according to Roberts and Gans (2008), is given in Table 6–4. BPPV affecting the anterior semicircular canal (ASC-BPPV) and multiple canals is much less common accounting for no more than 5% of cases (Moon et al., 2006; De la Meilleur et al., 1996).

As described above, the prevalence and clinical presentation of BPPV is well known, yet the condition often goes undiagnosed or is treated inappropriately. Also, because BPPV represents a "mechanical" impairment in the vestibular end organ, the condition may disappear spontaneously and go through long periods of remission. It is important that clinicians in the balance clinic work closely with the referring professional in order to identify and treat patients with BPPV in a timely and appropriate manner.

Pathophysiology

Our understanding of the pathophysiologic mechanism of BPPV has evolved significantly over the past 40 years. The initial pathophysiologic mechanism for BPPV was provided by Harold Schuknecht (1962). Using photomicrographs, he uncovered basophilic particles that had attached to the cupula. He proposed that these densities were displaced otoconia from the utricular maculae and the primary source of BPPV (Schuknecht, 1969; Schuknecht & Ruby, 1973). The cupula is a gelatinous mass housed in the ampullated end of each SCC. The role of the cupula is to transduce angular head accelerations into increases or decreases in neural firing rate. The cupula is normally a neutrally buoyant structure due to the fact that it has the same specific gravity as the surrounding endolymph. When the head is subjected to acceleration, the hydrodynamic pressure from the endolymph distorts the cupula and triggers a response from the hair cells embedded in the base.

Table 6–4. Incidence of Benign Paroxysmal Positional Vertigo Among Semicircular Canals

Study	Number	PC	HC	AC
Herdman, Tusa, & Clendaniel (1994)	59	63.6	1.3	11.7
Fife (1998)	424	91	6	3
Wolf, Boyev, Manokey, & Mattox (1999)	107	95.3	1.9	2.8
Honrubia, Baloh, Harris, & Jacobson (1999)	292	93.5	5.1	1.4
Ruckenstein (2001)	86	96.5	2.3	1.2
Korres & Balatsouras (2004)	122	90.2	8.2	1.6
Cakir et al. (2006)	169	85.2	11.8	1.2
Jackson, Morgan, Fletcher, & Krueger (2007)	260	66.9	11.9	21.2

PC posterior canal; *HC* horizontal canal; *AC* anterior canal
Source: From Roberts & Gans (2008, p. 181)

This displacement of the cupula and shearing of the hair cells generates a neural code associated with movement. If the acceleration continues, the viscoelastic nature of the cupula returns it to its original position; however, when otoconial debris is displaced from the utricle it can adhere to the cupula and change its density. This creates a situation where a sustained movement in the plane of the impaired canal causes the cupula to remain in a position where the debris exerts a force that keeps it deflected toward the earth. The description of this series of events led Schuknecht to coin the term "cupulolithiasis." This theory persisted until the early 1990s and was the model used to develop the early Cawthorne and Brandt-Daroff treatments (Cawthorne, 1944; Brandt & Daroff, 1980). At the time of this writing it continues to be one of the two prevailing pathophysiologic mechanisms of BPPV.

Approximately 30 years later, John Epley (1992) postulated the "canalithiasis" theory of BPPV based on models of the labyrinth he developed. He set forth that the characteristic symptoms of BPPV (i.e., the fatigability and latency of the response) were more consistent with loose particles floating in the canals rather than attached to the cupula as Schuknecht had earlier proposed. This theory also supported the observed findings described by Dix and Hallpike (1952). In the very

same year, Parnes and McClure (1992), located at the University of London in Ontario, observed free-floating particles in the endolymphatic space of a patient undergoing a posterior semicircular canal (PSC) fenestration procedure. The particulate matter found in the PSC was hypothesized to be otoliths (which normally rest on the otolith membrane of the utricle and saccule) that had migrated from the utricular maculae and entered the PSC by way of the ductus reuniens. Otoliths (or canaliths if they have become free floating in the canal) are "heavier" than the surrounding endolymph. This means that, when at rest, the otoliths "sink" to the lowest level of the gravitational vector. When the head changes position the otolith debris also changes position en masse and in so doing displaces the endolymph. The endolymph displacement deflects the cupula (which is attached to the cristae) that normally occurs when the head is moving and, in so doing, sends a set of signals to the brain that normally would occur if the person were rotating. Parnes and McClure suggested that once enough of these otoliths accumulate in the PSC, they would form a large enough mass that would alter the physiologic characteristics of fluid motion in the SCCs. The authors added further support to this concept of free-floating particles by observing and documenting the symptoms of patients with BPPV.

These observations of the pathophysiology provided by Parnes and McClure along with Epley's models of the vestibular system provided the understanding that led to the development of the current canalith repositioning procedures (CRP) to treat patients with BPPV (Epley, 1992; Parnes & Price-Jones, 1993). The cupulolithiasis and canalithiasis pathophysiologic mechanisms as proposed by Schuknecht and Epley, respectively, continue to be the two primary theories explaining BPPV. Canalithiasis has been reported to be far more common than cupulolithiasis (Parnes et al., 2003).

Canalithiasis

Figures 6–5 and 6–6 illustrate how free-floating densities known as "canaliths" have been theorized to create aberrant endolymphatic flow with changes in the position of the head. In this set of figures, the patient is sitting supine and the canaliths have collected in the bottom of the PSC. When the head is turned and the patient is laid in the supine position (e.g., Dix-Hallpike maneuver), the right PSC and ASCs are placed in a position where the canaliths can fall. Because the canaliths are denser than the surrounding endolymph, they are under the influence of gravity and will begin to drop. Endolymph is very thick and there is a short delay between the movement of the particles and when gravity begins to act on them. Once the canaliths begin to settle in the canal, the hydrodynamic drag caused by the movement induces endolymph flow and consequently deflects the cupula (Figure 6–6). In the vertical canals, the stereocilia in the cupula are oriented away from the utricle, and endolymph flow created by the falling densities when the patient is placed in the supine position creates an excitatory response from the vestibulo-ocular reflex (VOR). Because the VOR is being activated and the patient is not moving, the perception by the patient is of vertigo. Once the canaliths have gravitated to the lowest point in the canal, endolymph flow stops, the cupula returns to its neutral position, the neural drive to the VOR returns to its tonic resting rate, and the perception of vertigo by the patient ceases (Parnes & McClure, 1992). When the patient is brought back to the sitting position, the canaliths again begin to

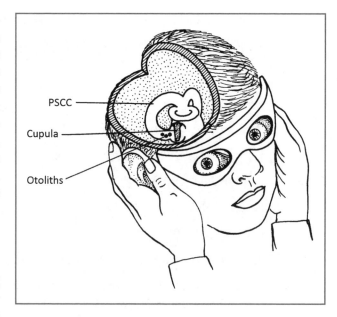

FIGURE 6–5. An illustration of canalithiasis. The particles are located in the posterior semicircular canal with the patient sitting. **PSCC** posterior semicircular canal. (Courtesy of Daniel Pender, adapted from Pender, 1992)

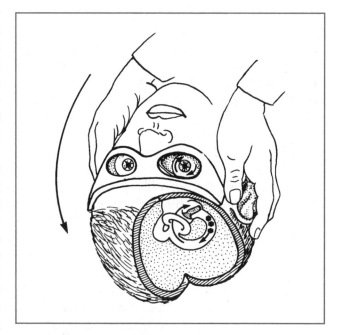

FIGURE 6–6. An illustration of canalithiasis. Following a provocative maneuver, the particles drop and trigger the vestibulo-ocular reflex. (Courtesy of Daniel Pender, adapted from Pender, 1992)

drop and in this instance the cupula is deflected in the opposite direction, generating an inhibitory response (typically smaller) from the VOR and a reversal in the perceived movement by the patient (i.e., the nystagmus beats in the opposite direction).

Cupulolithiasis

In the cupulolithiasis variant of BPPV, the displaced otoliths are attached to the cupula, causing it to become heavier and therefore sensitive to gravity. This condition is less common than the canalithiasis type and is more resistant to treatment. The response patterns (direction of the nystagmus) are very similar to those of canalithiasis (described above), but the characteristics of the responses can be different. For example, because the otoliths are attached directly to the cupula, the response is often immediate (no latent period) (Figure 6–7). Additionally, in cases of cupulolithiasis the nystagmus may continue for a longer time if the head is maintained in a provocative position.

Diagnosis

The correct diagnosis of BPPV and the identification of the canal(s) that are involved are dependent on the clinician being able to interpret the pattern of responses that occur following the movement of the patient into a position that provokes his or her vertigo. There are several maneuvers that have been designed to orient each SCC into a position where any displaced otoconia will be subject to the pull of gravity and stimulate the canal. However, it is not enough to just provoke the vertigo. The examiner must also have a thorough understanding of the semicircular canal ocular reflexes in order to correctly characterize the nystagmus and identify the location of the displaced particles. Each SCC is connected to a pair of eye muscles in such a way that when the canal is stimulated, the eyes move in the plane of that canal (Figure 6–8). This is the premise of Ewald's first law, which states that the direction of the nystagmus should match the anatomic axis of the SCC that is stimulated (Ewald, 1892). These disynaptic connections between the SCCs and the eyes allow the clinician

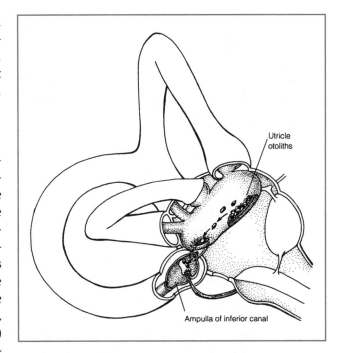

FIGURE 6–7. An illustration of cupulolithiasis affecting the posterior semicircular canal. (Courtesy of Daniel Pender, adapted from Pender, 1992)

to accurately identify the location of the canaliths and form a correct treatment plan. Table 6–5 summarizes the excitatory actions of each of the canals and the associated nystagmus.

Posterior Canal BPPV

The Dix-Hallpike maneuver is the gold standard for identifying PSC-BPPV (Dix & Hallpike, 1952). Before the maneuver is performed, the patients should be counseled regarding how they will be moved during the positioning and that they may experience some dizziness. It is important to reassure the patient that the dizziness will be transient (less than 60 s). The traditional Dix-Hallpike maneuver begins with the patient sitting on the exam table and the head turned 45° from midline toward the side that is being assessed. With the neck supported, the examiner guides the patient back into the supine position with the head hyperextended approximately 30° below the horizontal plane. The clinician should be in a position where the patient's eyes can be clearly viewed. A positive

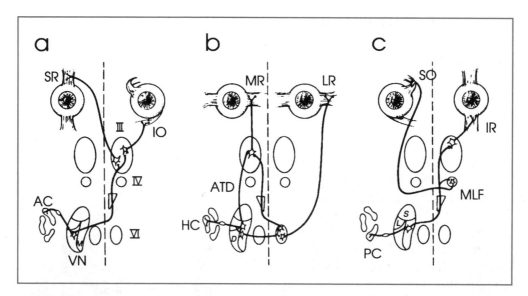

FIGURE 6–8. A–C. The excitatory connections between the semicircular canals and the extraocular eye muscles. **SR** superior rectus; **AC** anterior canal; **VN** vestibular nucleus; **IO** inferior oblique; **MR** medial rectus; **LR** lateral rectus; **ATD** ; **HC** horizontal canal; **SO** superior oblique; **IR** inferior rectus; **MLF** medial longitudinal fasciculus; **PC** posterior canal. *Roman numerals* indicate cranial nerves. (From Baloh & Kerber, 2011)

Table 6–5. Excitatory Actions of Each of the Canals and the Associated Nystagmus

Canal	Eye Muscles Activated	Associated Nystagmus (Fast Phase)
Posterior	Ipsilateral superior oblique Contralateral inferior rectus	Torsional/up-beating
Horizontal	Ipsilateral medial rectus Contralateral lateral rectus	Horizontal
Anterior	Ipsilateral superior rectus Contralateral inferior oblique	Torsional/down-beating

response is indicated by vertigo and a torsional up-beating nystagmus in the supine position directed toward the dependent ear (Figure 6–9). The characteristics of PSC BPPV are described in Table 6–6 and an example of a VNG recording is presented in Figure 6–10. Before performing the Dix-Hallpike maneuver, the examiner should have a thorough understanding of the patient's medical history. For instance, in order to avoid injuring the patient, caution should be exercised when assessing patients presenting with a history of vascular or orthopedic disorders (e.g., vertebro-basilar insufficiency, cervical spondylosis, kyphoscoliosis, or cervical radiculopathy). In patients where hyperextension of the neck is contraindicated, a modified procedure known as the side-lying maneuver is an alternative technique to the Dix-Hallpike maneuver to assess the PSC (Herdman & Tusa, 1996). Humphriss, Baguley, Sparkes, Peerman, & Moffat (2003) compared the sensitivity of the Dix-Hallpike maneuver to the side-lying maneuver for the identification of PSC-BPPV. The investigators reported no significant difference between the two assessments.

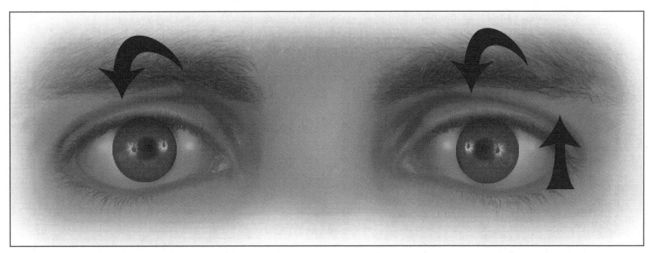

A

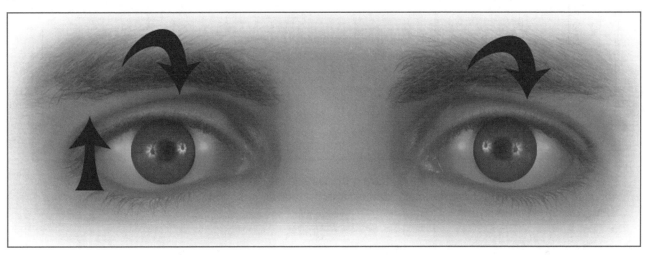

B

FIGURE 6–9. A. Eye movements from a right-side posterior semicircular canal benign paroxysmal positional vertigo. Up-beating nystagmus with a torsional component to the right when the head is placed in the head-down right position. Straight *arrows* indicate the vertical direction of the fast phase of the nystagmus. Curved *arrows* indicate the torsional direction of the fast phase of the nystagmus. **B.** Eye movements from a left-side posterior semicircular canal benign paroxysmal positional vertigo. Up-beating nystagmus with a torsional component to the left when the head is placed in the head-down left position. Straight *arrows* indicate the vertical direction of the fast phase of the nystagmus. Curved *arrows* indicate the torsional direction of the fast phase of the nystagmus.

Table 6–6. Characteristics of Posterior Semicircular Canal Benign Paroxysmal Positioning Vertigo

Duration	Usually less than 40 s
Direction change	Down-beating when returning to the sitting position
Fatigability	Intensity reduces when the maneuver is repeated
Temporal course	Initial increase in intensity and then slowly declines
Direction of nystagmus	Torsional/up-beating when placed in the initial provocative position

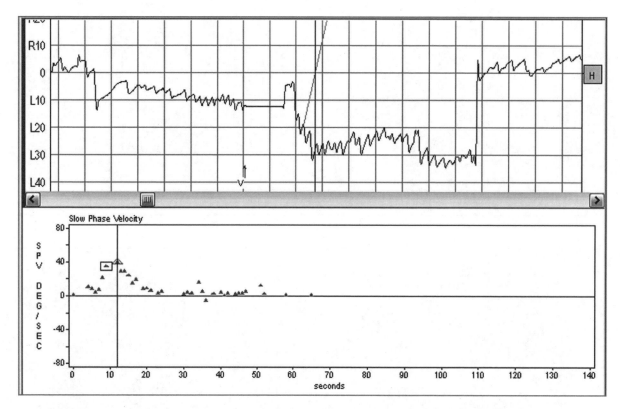

FIGURE 6–10. Up-beating nystagmus during the Dix-Hallpike maneuver in a patient with canalithiasis affecting the right posterior semicircular canal. Note the abrupt onset and then decline of the response. **SPV** slow-phase velocity.

Instruction Set Delivered to Patient Prior to the Maneuver

The instructions to be given to the patient are as follows:

> In just a moment we are going to make believe you are laying down in bed with your head turned to the right (or left). I would like you to cross your arms over your chest like this (demonstrate), turn your head to the right (or left), and then I will count to three. On three, I want you to let me guide you back so that you are laying on your back with your head just a bit over the edge of the table. We will stay there for about half a minute. It is critical that you keep your eyes open all of this time. You may or may not have a sensation of movement when you lay down. If you do, it is likely that your eyes will be moving a little bit and how they move tells us which maneuver we need to do to rid you of this positional vertigo. So no matter what sensation you experience, please keep your eyes wide open. Are you

ready? I will count to 3 and on 3 we will lay back: 1—2—3.

Technique for the Dix-Hallpike Maneuver

The technique for the Dix-Hallpike maneuver is as follows:

1. The patient begins the maneuver seated in the upright position and the clinician stands on the side that is to be tested. It is important to ensure that the patient is oriented so that when they are put into the supine position the head will hang off the edge of the table.
2. The clinician should have the patient turn his head 45° toward the examiner and make sure that the hands are placed in a position where the neck is supported. Before the maneuver is initiated, patients should be instructed to make sure that they keep their eyes open.

3. The examiner lays the patient back and extends the patient's head approximately 30° below the horizontal plane.
4. The examiner observes the patient's eyes for 30 s.
5. The nystagmus should be up-beating and torsional directed toward the dependent ear. After the nystagmus stops, the patient should be returned to the upright position. Once the patient is in the upright position, the patient will often experience dizziness again and the nystagmus should reverse direction.
6. The Dix-Hallpike maneuver should then be repeated for the other side, and complete the same series of steps as outlined above (Figure 6–11).

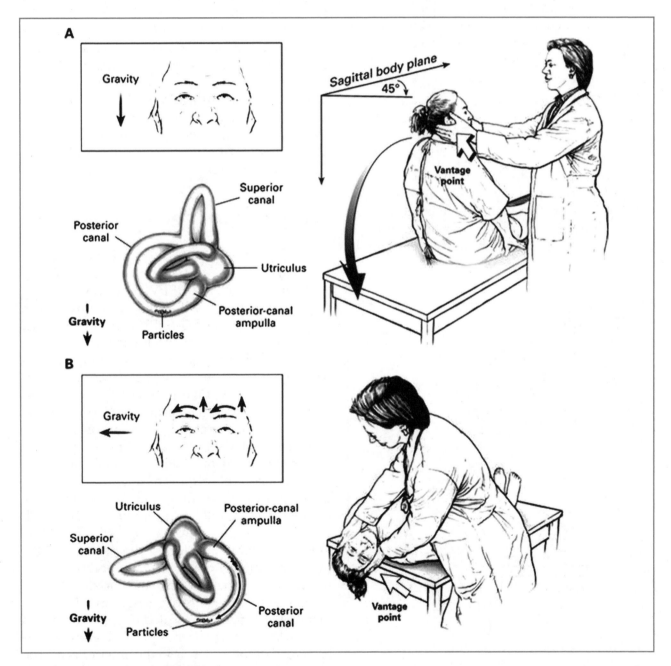

FIGURE 6–11. **A** and **B.** Illustration of the technique of the Dix-Hallpike maneuver to the right. **A.** The clinician stands on the right side, rotates the patient's head 45°, and supports the neck. **B.** The patient is then moved into a supine right-ear-down position with the head hyperextended and eyes open. (From Bhattacharyya et al., 2008)

Technique for the Side-Lying Test

The technique for the side-lying test is as follows:

1. The patient is seated on the exam table facing the clinician.
2. The head is turned 45° away from the ear that is intended to be assessed.
3. While maintaining the head position the patient is quickly moved to the side-lying position (avoid hyperextension) and the legs are brought up onto the exam table.
4. This position is held for approximately 30 s.
5. Patient is returned to the seated position (Figure 6–12).

Mechanism

The Dix-Hallpike and side-lying maneuvers place the posterior canal in the vertical plane (aligned with earth vertical), causing the canaliths to drop when the head is hung 30° over the end of the exam table. The orientation of the stereocilia in the posterior canals is such that when the otoliths gravitate, they create ampullopetal flow of the endolymph and deflect the cupula. This induces an excitatory response from the canal and activates the VOR. The VOR contracts the ipsilateral superior oblique and contralateral inferior rectus extraocular muscles and a consequent nystagmus is generated. The slow phases of the nystagmus are directed in such a way as to drive the eyes downward with intorsion of the eye toward the lower ear and extorsion of the upper eye. The upper poles of the eyes beat up and toward the dependent ear during the fast corrective phase of the nystagmus (torsional up-beating). Upon sitting, the canaliths again move, creating endolymph flow in the opposite direction and pressure on the cupula (ampullofugal), which generates a nystagmus that beats in the opposite direction (i.e., down-beating).

Horizontal Canal BPPV

In contrast to PSC-BPPV, there are two forms of horizontal semicircular canal BPPV (HSC-BPPV). Each variant of HSC-BPPV produces different responses that are used to design the treatment. The classic sign of HSC-BPPV is nystagmus that is purely horizontal with no torsional component evoked with lateral head turns in the supine position. The most common type of HSC-BPPV generates a nystagmus with the fast phase directed toward the ground (i.e., geotropic) (Figure 6–13). Figure 6–14 illustrates a VNG recording of a patient with HSC-BPPV that generates a geotropic response with lateral head turns. HSC-BPPV can also produce apogeotropic nystagmus (fast phase directed away from the ground) (Figure 6–15). Figure 6–16 is a VNG recording of a patient with HSC-BPPV that produces apogeotropic nystagmus with lateral head turns. The direction of the nystagmus affords the clinician the ability to localize where the canaliths are in the horizontal canal. In other words, geotropic nystagmus indicates that there are particles located in posterior arm of the HSC, whereas apogeotropic nystagmus is suggestive of otolithic debris in the anterior arm. The test for diagnosing HSC-BPPV is the supine head-roll maneuver (i.e., Pagnini-McClure maneuver).

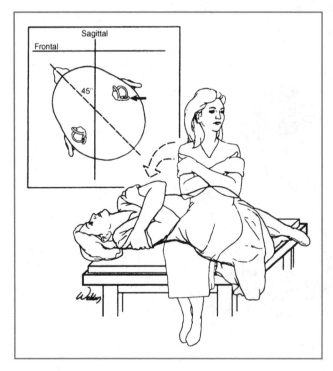

FIGURE 6–12. Illustration of the side-lying maneuver. (From Cohen, 2004)

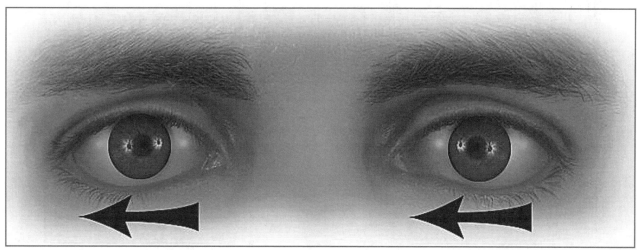

A

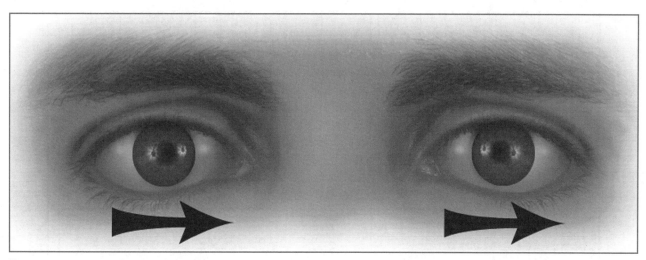

B

FIGURE 6–13. **A.** Eye movements from a right-side horizontal semicircular canal (right posterior arm) benign paroxysmal positional vertigo. Horizontal nystagmus with stronger response when the head is turned to the right and the right ear is down (geotropic). *Arrows* indicate fast phase of the nystagmus. **B.** Eye movements from a left-side horizontal semicircular canal (left posterior arm) benign paroxysmal positional vertigo. Horizontal nystagmus with stronger response when the head is turned to the left and the left ear is down (geotropic). *Arrows* indicate fast phase of the nystagmus.

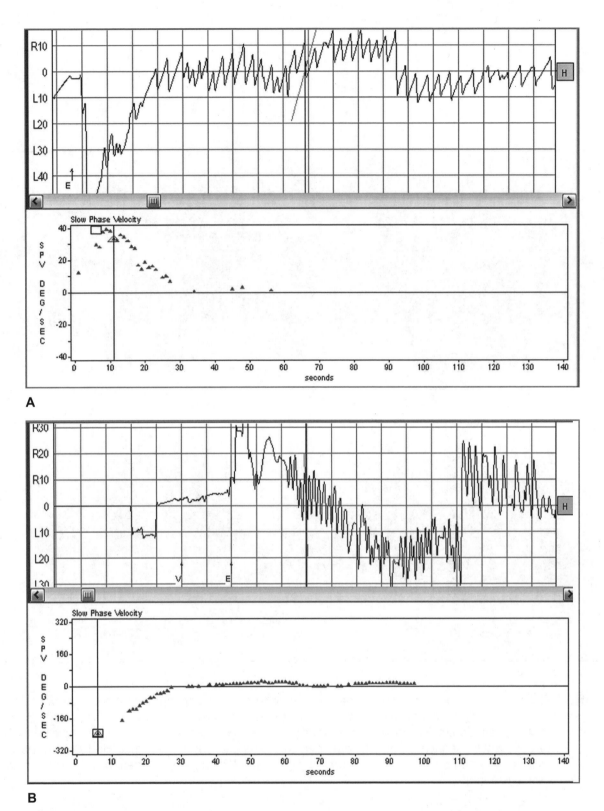

FIGURE 6–14. A. Horizontal nystagmus during the roll maneuver to the left in a patient with canalithiasis affecting the right lateral semicircular canal. The particles are located in the posterior arm. Note that the response is smaller than the response from the right (affected side). **SPV** slow-phase velocity. **B.** Horizontal nystagmus during the roll maneuver to the right in a patient with canalithiasis affecting the right lateral semicircular canal. The particles are located in the posterior arm. Note that the response is larger than the response from the left (unaffected side). **SPV** slow-phase velocity.

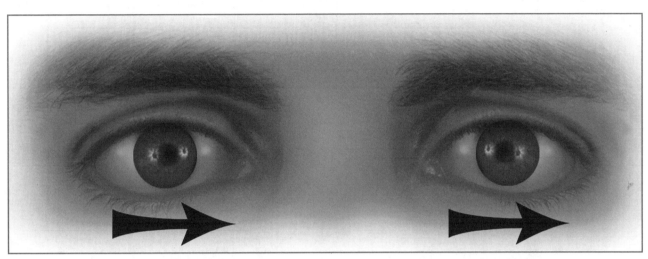

A

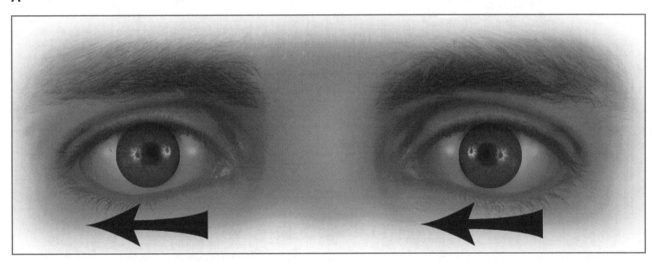

B

FIGURE 6–15. **A.** Eye movements from a right-side horizontal semicircular canal (right anterior arm) benign paroxysmal positional vertigo. Left-beating horizontal nystagmus is observed with a weaker response when the head is turned to the right and the right ear is down (apogeotropic). *Arrows* indicate fast phase of the nystagmus. **B.** Eye movements from a left-side horizontal semicircular canal (left anterior arm) benign paroxysmal positional vertigo. Right-beating horizontal nystagmus is observed with a weaker response when the head is turned to the left and the left ear is down (apogeotropic). *Arrows* indicate fast phase of the nystagmus.

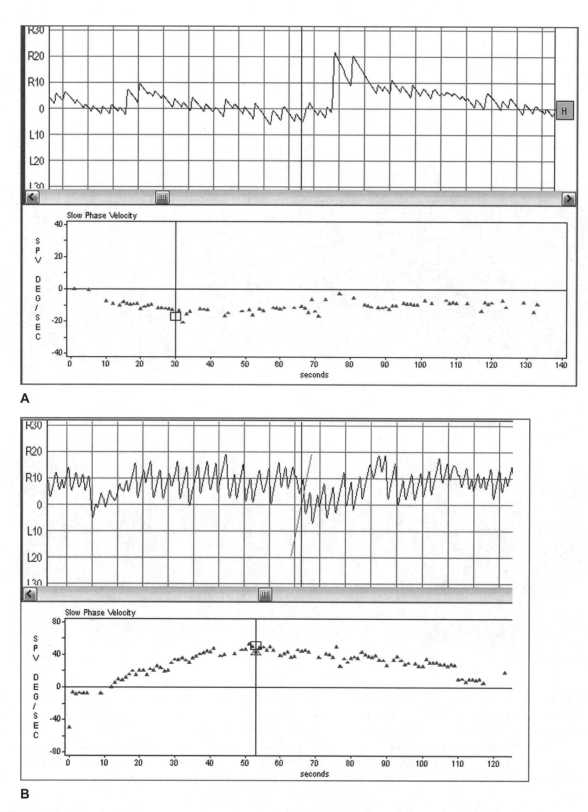

FIGURE 6–16. **A.** Horizontal apogeotropic nystagmus during the roll maneuver to the left in a patient with cana-lithiasis affecting the left lateral semicircular canal. The particles are located in the left anterior arm of the horizontal canal. Note that the response is smaller than the response from the right (unaffected side). **SPV** slow-phase velocity. **B.** Horizontal apogeotropic nystagmus during the roll maneuver to the right in a patient with canalithiasis affecting the left lateral semicircular canal. The particles are located in the left anterior arm of the horizontal canal. Note that the response is larger than the response from the left (affected side). **SPV** slow-phase velocity.

This assessment consists of the examiner placing the patient in the supine position on an exam table with the head elevated approximately 30° (i.e., the same position used for caloric testing) and rotating it to the right and left. The supine roll test provides two critical pieces of information that the examiner later uses to treat the disorder. First, the maneuver enables the clinician to identify the affected side (i.e., right or left). Localization of the affected ear is based on a comparison of the intensity of the nystagmus between the left and right head turns. This is based on Ewald's second law, which sets forth that excitation (ampullopetal flow of endolymph) of the HSC (i.e., horizontal) produces a more robust (nystagmus) response than inhibition (ampullofugal flow of endolymph) of the HSC (Ewald, 1892); however, there are occasionally patients in whom the right and left head turns produce symmetric responses making it difficult to identify the affected side. Reasons for this may include a different angle with which the supine head roll is done from left to right or where the otolithic mass is positioned when the head is rolled (Strupp, Brandt, & Steddin, 1995). In these cases, there are alternative techniques that can be employed to determine which ear is impaired (e.g., the "bow and lean" test). Second, the direction of the nystagmus (i.e., geotropic or apogeotropic) that is provoked localizes where the otolithic debris resides in the HSC (i.e., anterior or posterior arm). A positive response is indicated by vertigo and nystagmus with lateral head turns, the characteristics of which are described in Table 6–7.

Instruction Set Delivered to Patient Prior to the Maneuver

The instructions given to the patient are as follows:

> In just a moment we are going to make believe you are turning your head side to side while laying in bed. I will count to three. On three, I want you to turn your head quickly all the way to the right and hold it there until I ask you to return it to the center. We will stay there for about half a minute. It is critical that you keep your eyes open all of this time. You may or may not have a sensation of movement after you turn your head. If you do, it is likely that your eyes will be moving a little bit and how they move tells us which maneuver we need to do to rid you of this positional vertigo. So no matter what sensation you experience, please keep your eyes wide open. Are you ready? I will count to 3 and on 3 we will lay back: 1—2—3.

Technique for the Supine Head-Roll Test

The technique for the supine head-roll test is as follows:

1. The patient is moved into the supine position with the head elevated 30° and then asked to rotate his head 90° to one side.
2. Following the head movement, the examiner should observe the patient's eyes for any

Table 6–7. Characteristics of Horizontal Semicircular Canal Benign Paroxysmal Positioning Vertigo

Duration	Usually less than 60 s
Direction change	Reverses direction on lateral head turns
Fatigability	Intensity reduces when the maneuver is repeated
Temporal course	Initial increase in intensity and then slowly declines
Direction of nystagmus	Linear–horizontal (can be geotropic or apogeotropic)

nystagmus for a period of 30 s. If nystagmus is observed, the direction and duration should be noted.

3. The head should be returned to the center (patient is facing up and forward) and held in this position until there is no longer any measurable nystagmus.
4. The head is rotated 90° to the opposite side and again the eyes should be observed for 30 s and the characteristics of any nystagmus noted (Figure 6–17).

Lateralizing the Impaired Ear Using the Supine Head-Roll Test

With geotropic nystagmus, the affected ear is presumed to be the side with the larger amplitude and the particles located in the posterior arm of the HSC. With apogeotropic nystagmus, the affected ear is presumed to be the side with the smaller amplitude and the particles located in the anterior arm of the HSC.

Technique for the "Bow and Lean" Test

The technique for the "bow and lean" test is as follows:

1. The supine roll test is performed and the nystagmus direction is noted (geotropic or apogeotropic).
2. The patient then sits on the exam table facing the clinician.
3. The patient is asked to bow his head 90° forward and the direction, amplitude, and duration of any nystagmus is recorded.
4. The patient tilts his head backward 45°, and again the characteristics of the nystagmus are documented.

Lateralizing the Impaired Ear Using the "Bow and Lean" Test

When the supine head-roll test generates geotropic nystagmus, the affected ear is the same as the

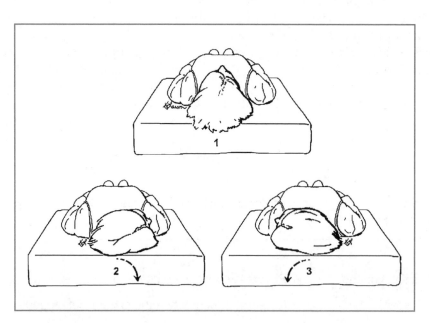

FIGURE 6–17. The supine roll maneuver (Pagnini-McClure maneuver), to the right and then left, is shown. (From Bhattacharyya et al., 2008)

direction of the fast phase of the bowing nystagmus and the opposite of the direction of the fast phase of the leaning nystagmus (Figure 6–18). When the supine head-roll test generates apogeotropic nystagmus, the affected ear is the opposite of the direction of the fast phase of bowing nystagmus and the same as the direction of the fast phase of the leaning nystagmus (Figure 6–19).

Mechanism

In order to treat HSC-BPPV, the canal where the particles are located must be determined. To accurately identify the affected canal requires that the examiner understand the biomechanics behind the various physiologic responses that occur when a patient has HSC-BPPV. When the head

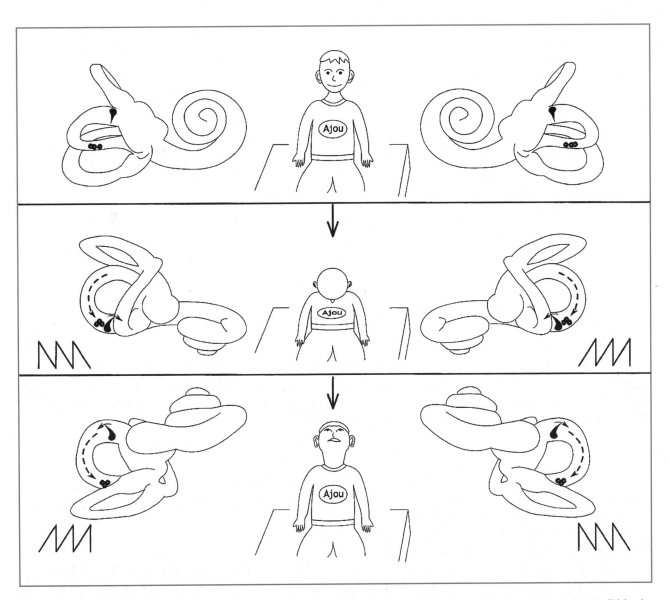

FIGURE 6–18. The "bow and lean" test for diagnosing the affected ear in cases of horizontal canal canalithiasis. The nystagmus beats in the same direction as the bowing nystagmus and the opposite direction of the leaning nystagmus. (From Choung et al., 2006)

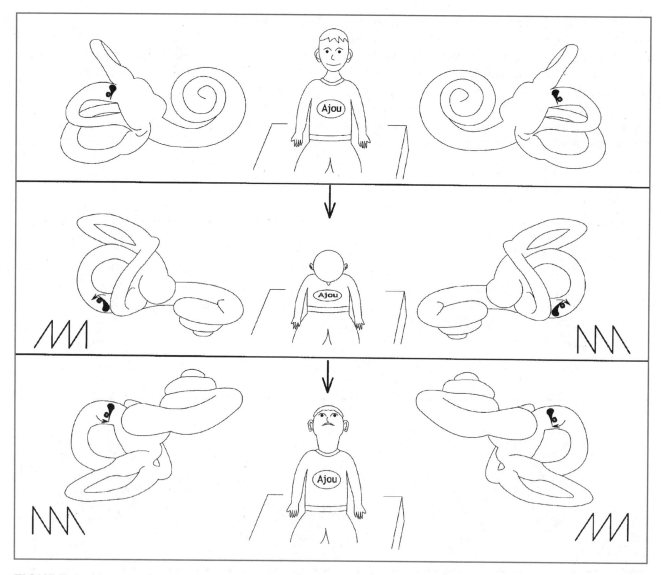

FIGURE 6–19. The "bow and lean" test for diagnosing the affected ear in cases of horizontal canal cupuloli-thiasis. In this instance, the nystagmus beats in the opposite direction as the bowing nystagmus and the same direction of the leaning nystagmus. (From Choung et al., 2006)

is moved, canaliths in the HSC cause the endo-lymph to move in a predictable way based on where they are located in the HSC. Ampullopetal flow of endolymph is excitatory and generates a larger response than ampullofugal flow, which is inhibitory (Ewald's second law). The clinician is able to identify the impaired canal by recording the direction and amplitude of the responses from the right and left and then comparing them. There are three patterns of HSC-BPPV: bilateral geotro-pic, bilateral apogeotropic that can be converted to bilateral geotropic, and bilateral apogeotropic that cannot be converted to bilateral geotropic.

Geotropic HSC

Geotropic HSC, a variant of HSC-BPPV, is the most common form and produces a bilateral geotropic nystagmus during lateral head turns (Caruso & Nuti, 2005). The pathophysiologic mechanism of the geotropic variant of HSC-BPPV is the presence of dislodged otoconia, most likely

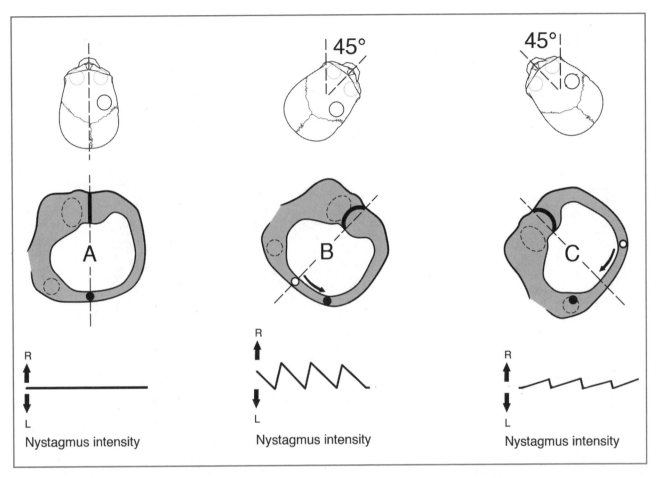

FIGURE 6–20. A–C. The mechanism of right-sided horizontal canal canalithiasis with the particles located in the posterior arm of the canal. **A.** Supine with no nystagmus. **B.** Head turn to the right generates a larger-amplitude right-beating nystagmus (geotropic). **C.** Head turn to the left generates a smaller left-beating nystagmus.

from the utricle, located in the posterior arm of the HSC (Figure 6–20A) (Nuti et al., 1992). The location of these particles is such that when the head is moved toward the affected ear, ampullopetal flow of the endolymph is induced and a corresponding vertigo and nystagmus occurs. When the head is turned toward the unaffected side, ampullofugal flow occurs in the affected canal, which again generates vertigo and a nystagmus that beats in the opposite direction. The reason for this is that when the is head turned toward the affected ear, the particles drop and move the endolymph in a way that produces an excitatory response resulting in a large-amplitude horizontal nystagmus with the fast component beating toward the ground (lower ear) (see Figure 6–20B). When the

head is turned in the opposite direction toward the unaffected side, the nystagmus will again be geotropic but smaller in amplitude due to the inhibitory action of the endolymph flow (Figure 6–20C).

Apogeotropic HSC

Apogeotropic nystagmus has been theorized to be attributed to particles located in the superior arm of the HSC. Casani et al. (2002) has reported the characteristics of two different types of apogeotropic HSC-BPPV. The first variant consists of otoliths attached to the cupula on the utricular side of the canal (Figure 6–21). The second type of apogeotropic HSC consists of debris on the canal side of

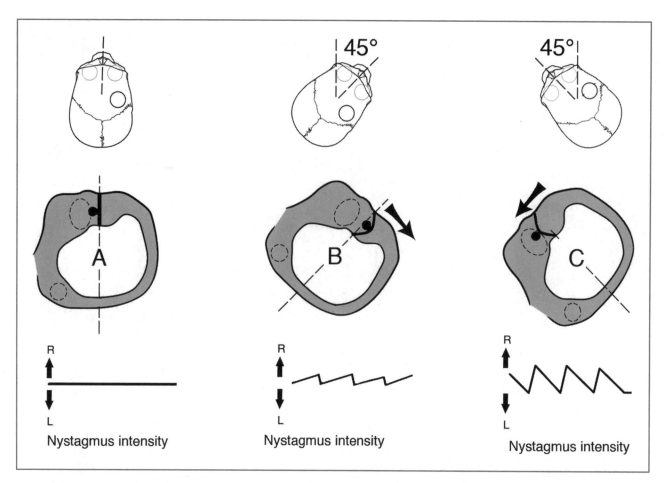

FIGURE 6–21. A–C. The mechanism of right-sided horizontal canal cupulolithiasis with the particles located on the utricular side of the cupula in the anterior arm of the canal. **A.** Supine with no nystagmus. **B.** Head turn to the right generates a smaller-amplitude left-beating nystagmus (apogeotropic). **C.** Head turn to the left generates a larger right-beating nystagmus.

the cupula (Figure 6–22). In cases of apogeotropic BPPV, when the head is turned in the direction of the unaffected ear, the canaliths either move (canalithiasis) and create endolymph flow or the cupula is weighted (cupulolithiasis) in such a way that the movement produces an ampullopetal (excitatory) deflection of the cupula. This generates an intense apogeotropic nystagmus. Conversely, a head turn toward the impaired ear causes the particles to deflect the cupula in an ampullofugal (inhibitory) manner resulting in the generation of an apogeotropic horizontal nystagmus that is less intense than when the head is turned toward the healthy side (Asprella Libonati, 2005; Han, Oh, & Kim, 2006; Koo, Moon, Shim, Moon, & Kim, 2006).

Anterior Canal BPPV

The assessment of the anterior semicircular canal (ASC) can be done using the traditional Dix-Hallpike maneuver described previously or a straight-back head-hanging maneuver. This has consistently been reported in the literature as one of the rarest forms of BPPV (Herdman & Tusa, 1996; Honrubia, Baloh, Harris, & Jacobson, 1999; Korres et al., 2002). Because of the vertical orientation of the ASC, it has been suggested that canaliths entering this canal often "self-clear" and migrate into either the vestibule or the PSC (Crevits, 2004). The anterior canal is oriented superiorly with its posterior arm connecting at the bottom of the common crus. While the Dix-

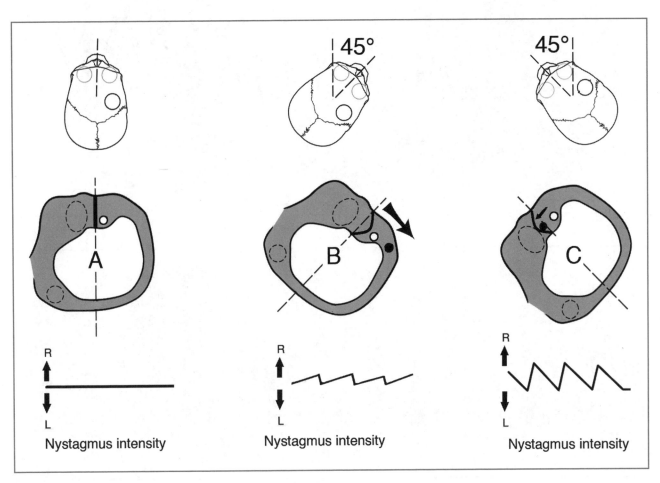

FIGURE 6–22. A–C. The mechanism of right-sided horizontal canal canalithiasis with the particles located on the canal side of the cupula in the anterior arm of the canal. **A.** supine with no nystagmus. **B.** Head turn to the right generates a smaller amplitude left-beating nystagmus (apogeotropic). **C.** Head turn to the left generates a larger right-beating nystagmus.

Hallpike is the maneuver of choice to evaluate a patient for PSC-BPPV, patients with ASC-BPPV will also commonly manifest nystagmus during this maneuver. The orientation of the ASC is such that when the head is rotated to the contralateral side 45° (as in the Dix-Hallpike maneuver), the ASC canal is oriented in the vertical plane. When the patient is placed in the head-hanging position, the ampulla is located anteriorly with the posterior arm located inferiorly. With this orientation of the ASC, the canaliths are subject to gravity and are able to drop posteriorly through the canal. A positive response is indicated by vertigo and a torsional/down-beating nystagmus in the supine position directed toward the dependent ear (Figure 6–23). (The characteristics of ASC-BPPV are

described in Table 6–8 and an example of a VNG recording is presented in Figure 6–24.) However, identifying the involved side can be challenging in patients with ASC-BPPV for two reasons. First, the torsional component is typically very small or absent and therefore is not as helpful for use in identifying the affected side as is the case with PSC-BPPV (Bertholon, Bronstein, Davies, Rudge, & Thilo, 2002). Second, anatomic differences in the ASC of patients can lead to the affected side producing larger responses in the ear oriented upward or the ear oriented downward (Crevits, 2004). For this reason, the straight-back head-hanging (SBHH) maneuver is a useful alternative to use for the assessment of ASC-BPPV (Yacovino et al., 2009). During the SBHH, the patient is laid

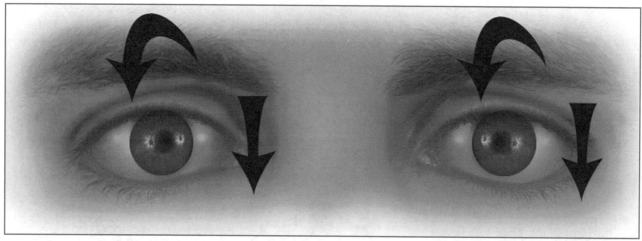

A

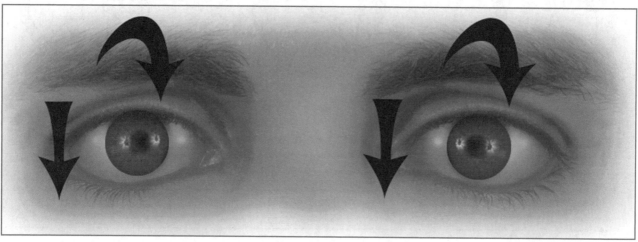

B

FIGURE 6–23. A. Eye movements from a right-side anterior semicircular canal benign paroxysmal positional vertigo. Down-beating nystagmus with a torsional component to the right when the head is placed in the head-down right position. Straight *arrows* indicate the vertical direction of the fast phase of the nystagmus. Curved *arrows* indicate the torsional direction of the fast phase of the nystagmus. **B.** Eye movements from a left-side anterior semicircular canal benign paroxysmal positional vertigo. Down-beating nystagmus with a torsional component to the left when the head is placed in the head-down left position. Straight *arrows* indicate the vertical direction of the fast phase of the nystagmus. Curved *arrows* indicate the torsional direction of the fast phase of the nystagmus.

Table 6–8. Characteristics of Anterior Semicircular Canal Benign Paroxysmal Positioning Vertigo

Duration	Usually less than 40 s
Direction change	Up-beating when returning to the sitting position
Fatigability	Intensity reduces when the maneuver is repeated
Temporal course	Initial increase in intensity and then slowly declines
Direction of nystagmus	Torsional/down-beating when placed in the provocative position (torsional component may be difficult to identify)

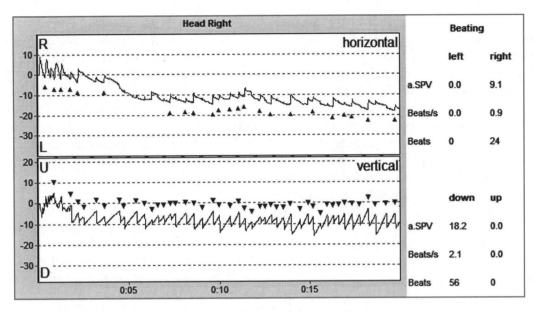

FIGURE 6–24. Down-beating nystagmus recorded during the Dix-Hallpike maneuver in a patient with canalithiasis affecting the right anterior semicircular canal.

straight back with the head hanging at least 30° below the horizontal plane, thereby aligning the posterior arm of the anterior canal with earth vertical (see Figure 6–33, Position 2). Using this technique provokes a more robust response than the Dix-Hallpike maneuver in most patients because of the ability to achieve a lower head position (Crevits, 2004). When the head is turned laterally 45° during the Dix-Hallpike maneuver, the ability to hang the head vertically is limited. The SBHH maneuver provides appropriate information regarding the disorder in order to prepare the patient for the treatment phase. The examiner must be vigilant to the presence of down-beating nystagmus, as it is also a strong central sign. Down-beating nystagmus must be observed very carefully to differentiate between ASC-BPPV and the more serious form that involves the cerebellum and/or brainstem. Down-beating nystagmus of central origin typically does not have a latent period before the response emerges, and it will not habituate.

Set of Instructions to the Patient

The instructions given to the patient are as follows:

> In just a moment we are going to make believe you are laying down in bed with your head hanging over the edge. I would like you to cross your arms over your chest like this (demonstrate), then I will count to three. On three, I want you to let me guide you back so that you are laying on your back with your head hanging over the edge of the table. We will stay there for about half a minute. It is critical that you keep your eyes open all of this time. You may or may not have a sensation of movement when you lay down. If you do, it is likely that your eyes will be moving a little bit and how they move tells us which maneuver we need to do to rid you of this positional vertigo. So no matter what sensation you experience please keep your eyes wide open. Are you ready? I will count to 3 and on 3 we will lay back: 1—2—3.

Technique for the Straight-Back Head-Hanging Maneuver

The technique for the SBHH maneuver is as follows:

1. The patient begins the maneuver seated in the upright position and the clinician sits or stands directly behind the patient. It is important to ensure that the patient is oriented so

that when he or she is put into the supine position, the head will hang off the edge of the table at least 30°. A thorough questioning of the patient regarding any cervical spine disorders should be undertaken before performing the maneuver.

2. The clinician should have the patient's head oriented straight ahead and ensure that the hands are placed in a position where the neck and head are supported. Before the maneuver is initiated, the patient should be instructed to make sure that he or she keeps his or her eyes open.

3. The examiner lays the patient back and extends the patient's head approximately 30° below the horizontal plane.

4. The examiner observes the patient's eyes for 30 s.

5. The nystagmus should be a primarily down-beating vertical eye movement with a slight torsional component. The torsional component may not always be evident.

6. After the nystagmus stops, the patient should be returned to the upright position. Once the patient is in the upright position, the patient often experiences dizziness again and the eyes reverse direction (up-beating nystagmus).

7. In ASC-BPPV it is important to document the latency, duration, and amplitude of the response. Locating the affected side for treatment is not as critical and is discussed in the treatment section of this chapter.

Mechanism

The ASC is positioned superiorly over the vestibule with the posterior arm oriented directly over the common crus and the utricle. In theory, any particles that migrate into the ASC should clear on their own when the patient lays supine; however, because of the geometry of the canal in some patients, it is thought that debris can accumulate in the anterior arm near the cupula. During the SBHH maneuver the head is hung over the end of an exam table aligning the posterior arm with the gravity vector. This allows gravity to act on the particles that are heavier than the surrounding endolymph causing them to move from the anterior arm through the posterior arm toward the common crus. The movement of the particles generates an ampullofugal deflection of the cupula (excitatory response) that activates the vestibulo-ocular reflex (VOR). The ASC sends projections through the brainstem to the contralateral inferior oblique and the ipsilateral superior rectus extraocular muscles. This excitatory activation of the ASC and corresponding contraction of the extraocular muscles produces a down-beating nystagmus.

When BPPV Has Been Diagnosed

The following is an example of how a patient could be counseled in lay terms regarding the mechanism of BPPV:

The inner ear organs of balance function like electrical generators, and there are 5 organs on each side for a total of 10. When you are sitting still, each inner ear system, the left and right ones, produce 1 million electrical signals per second. When the brain receives 1 million signals per second from each side, that is an electrical code that tells the brain you are sitting still. When you turn your head to the right, the electricity from the right inner ear goes up and the electricity from the left inner ear goes down. "High right" and "low left" is an electrical code that tells the brain you are turning your head to the right. If you turn your head to the left, the opposite happens. The electricity from the left inner ear goes up and the right inner ear goes down. "High left" and "low right" is an electrical code that tells the brain you are turning your head to the left. Now if you are sitting still and instead of the brain receiving equal electricity from each side it actually receives low electricity from the left side because disease has damaged the left inner ear, well, that is the code the brain normally receives when the head is turning toward the right (high right, low left). The brain then makes you feel like you are turning. So when you feel like you are moving and are not, that usually means that, at least for a period of time, the electrical output from one of the inner ears has either temporarily or permanently been reduced and the sensation you get because of that change is called "vertigo."

Now let's look a little closer at the organs in the inner ear that produce the electricity.

Three of the generators are located in half-circles filled with fluid. Since they are half-circles, call these things semicircular canals. Inside each one there is a device that is like gelatin and it "bends" when fluid pushes up against it. It is the bending of this device by the fluid that makes the electricity go up or down. The device moves when we turn our heads. The last two generators look a little different. They are made of calcium crystals that sit in a "net." Nerve fibers pass through the net up to the crystals. Just like gravel at the bottom of an aquarium would "shift" if we shook an aquarium back and forth or side to side, in the same way the "gravel" in the inner ear shifts from side to side if we accelerate or decelerate in a car or go up and down in an elevator. It is the shifting of the calcium crystals (the "gravel"), over the nerve endings that changes the electrical pattern coming from these devices that tells the brain what direction we are moving.

For various reasons, about which we are still not completely clear, these crystals can leave the "net" that normally holds them in place and drift to the semicircular canal system where they cause trouble. The crystals tend to clump together. If they are in the semicircular canal that reacts to forward and backward movement and you tip your head back at just the right angle, since the crystals are heavier than the inner ear fluid they will sink in the semicircular canal pushing the fluid ahead of them and bending the device in the semicircular canal that creates electricity. The result is that the sinking of the crystals in the semicircular canal produces the same electrical code that happens when we are turning, and that is the sensation we get. We call this positional vertigo because it occurs when we change position of the head or head and body together. It is the most common form of vertigo we see in the clinic, and since almost all of the time it does not mean that the person has a serious disease, it is referred to as "benign," "paroxysmal" because the vertigo sensation is big, "positional vertigo" because it occurs when we change the position of the head, or head and body together. We abbreviate this condition as "BPPV."

So, how do we get rid of this problem? Well, we can get rid of the problem if we can find a way to move or "reposition" the crystals to a different part of the inner ear where they cannot cause trouble. There are many differ-ent types of "repositioning maneuvers" that have been invented to do just that and they are referred to as "particle repositioning maneuvers" or "canalith repositioning maneuvers." The one that we choose for you will be customized for which semicircular canal we think the crystals are in.

TREATMENT OF BENIGN PAROXYSMAL POSITIONING VERTIGO

In many instances, BPPV self-remits with no intervention or treatment (Imai et al., 2005); however, some patients seek treatment before the BPPV resolves on its own. In these cases the clinician can treat the BPPV in the office at the time of the VNG/ENG. The treatment of BPPV is accomplished by using simple and effective maneuvers or exercises designed to move otoconial debris out of the impaired canal(s) and into the utricle where they do not generate aberrant canal responses. The two primary types of treatment that are discussed in the following section are liberatory maneuvers (e.g., Semont) and canalith repositioning procedures (CRP). The purpose of these techniques is to use a set of specific head positions that are based on the anatomy of the vestibular system to dislodge the displaced mass of otolithic debris and move it into a safe part of the end organ. When a treatment is successful, the symptoms of BPPV are resolved because the mass no longer creates abnormal endolymph flow and cupular displacement during head movements.

Posterior Semicircular Canal BPPV

The two most commonly reported CRP treatments for PSC canalithiasis are the modified Epley and Semont maneuvers (Epley, 1992; Semont, Freyss, & Vitte, 1988). Most CRP treatments of PSC-BPPV are based to some degree on Epley's original description of the treatment, with some modifications (Epley, 1992; Parnes & Price-Jones, 1993); however, there are occasions where the clinician encounters a patient who is unable to be treated using the conventional CRP (i.e., shoulder injury or in the morbidly obese). In such cases the Semont maneuver is an excellent alternative because it has been shown to have a similar efficacy when it comes to treating PSC-BPPV (Cohen & Kimball, 2005; Herdman, Tusa, Zee, Proctor, & Mattox, 1993; Cohen & Jerabeck, 1999; Salvinelli et al., 2004).

Modified Canalith Repositioning Procedure for PSC-BPPV

The modified CRP for PSC-BPPV is as follows (Figure 6–25):

1. The patient is placed in the upright position with the head turned 45° toward the affected ear (the ear that was positive on the Dix-Hall-pike testing).
2. The patient is rapidly laid back to the supine head-hanging position, which is maintained for approximately 90 s, starting when the sensation of vertigo has stopped.
3. The head is turned 90° toward the other (unaffected) side and held for approximately 90 s, starting when the sensation of vertigo has stopped.
4. Following this rotation, the head is turned a further 90° (usually necessitating the patient's body to also move from the supine position to the lateral decubitus position) such that the patient's head is nearly in the face-down position (i.e., nose pointing toward the ground). This position is also held for 90 s, starting when the sensation of vertigo has stopped.
5. The patient is then brought into the upright sitting position, completing the maneuver.

Semont Maneuver for Treatment of Right-Sided BPPV

The procedure for the Semont maneuver for the treatment of right-sided BPPV (Figure 6–26) is as follows:

1. The patient is seated on the examination table with legs hanging over the side.

2. The patient's head is rotated 45° toward the unaffected side.
3. While maintaining the head position the patient is quickly moved to the side-lying position.
4. This position is held for approximately 90 s, and then the patient is rapidly moved to the opposite side-lying position without pausing in the sitting position and without changing the head position relative to the shoulder.
5. This position is maintained for 90 s and then the patient gradually resumes the upright sitting position.

Treatment of Geotropic HSC-BPPV

The geotropic form of HSC-BPPV has been associated with the presence of canaliths in the posterior (nonampullar) arm. The treatment of this variant involves moving otolithic material from the posterior arm of the HSC into the vestibule. At the time of this writing there is no consensus in the literature regarding the "best" treatment for HSC-BPPV; however, there are two primary canalith repositioning (CRP) methods that have been thoroughly reported. The first method involves positioning the patient in the supine position and then rotating the head and body 270–360° (Lempert, 1994; Casani et al., 2002). These types of treatments have been referred to as "roll maneuvers" ("log" or "barbeque") and use gravity to move the canaliths in an ampullofugal direction until they reach the vestibule. A second type of CRP has been proposed by Asprella Libonati et al. (2005). This is a liberatory maneuver that has been reported to be successful in treating geotropic HSC-BPPV and has been praised in the literature for both its simplicity and success in treatment.

One reported way to increase the success rate of each of the above CRPs is to employ a technique known in the literature as "forced prolonged positioning" (FPP) (Nuti, Agus, Barbieri, & Passali, 1998; Casani et al., 2002). This method involves having the patient lay on the healthy side for approximately 12 hours (Vannucchi, Giannoni, & Pagnini, 1997; Parnes et al., 2003). Laying on the healthy side aligns the HSC in a manner that subjects it to the pull of gravity

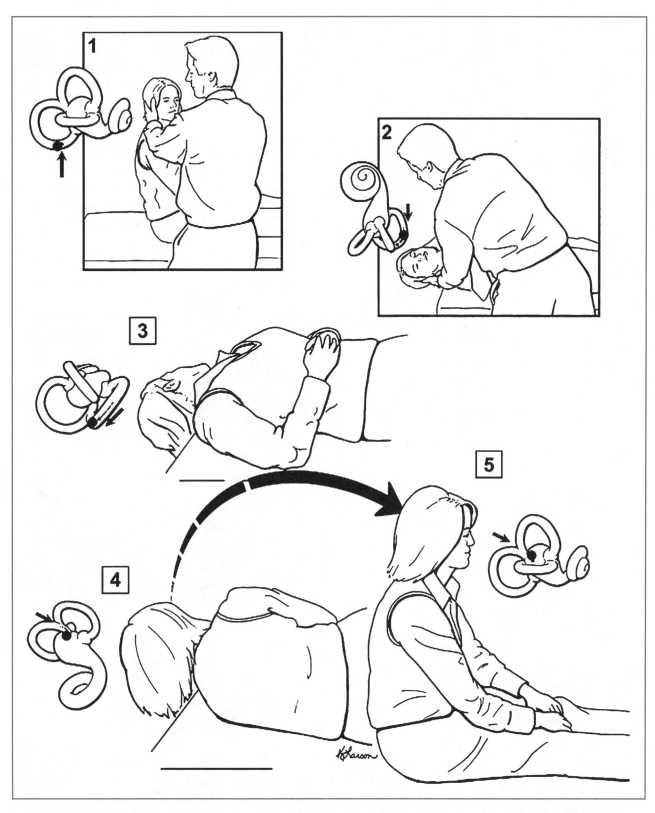

FIGURE 6–25. Illustration of the canalith repositioning procedure (modified Epley maneuver) to treat right posterior semicircular canal benign paroxysmal positioning vertigo (BPPV). (From Bhattacharyya et al., 2008)

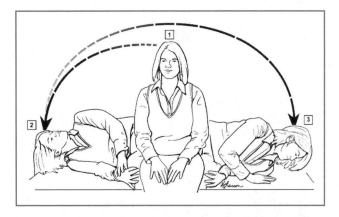

FIGURE 6–26. Illustration of the Semont maneuver used to treat right-sided BPPV. (From Bhattacharyya et al., 2008)

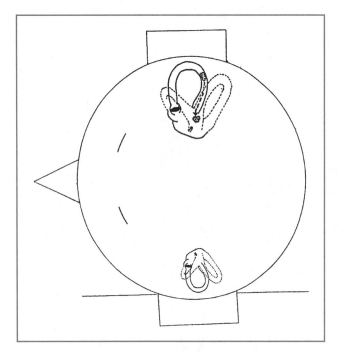

FIGURE 6–27. The "forced prolonged position" for a patient with right-sided horizontal canal BPPV. Note how the otolithic debris moves out of the horizontal canal and into the vestibule. (From Vannucchi et al., 1997)

(Figure 6–27). The patient maintains this position for approximately 12 hours the night following the CRP (Parnes et al., 2003). Several reports suggest the use of FPP in combination with canalith repositioning maneuvers in order to increase the success rate of treatment. It is also noteworthy that

in patients who are unable to undergo a CRP (e.g., patients who experience severe nausea during the maneuvers), the FPP can be used in isolation with a high degree of success (Chiou, Lee, Tsai, Yu, & Lee, 2005).

Roll Canalith Repositioning Maneuver

The procedure for the roll canalith repositioning maneuver (Figure 6–28) (Casani, Vannucci, Fattori, & Berrettini, 2002) is as follows:

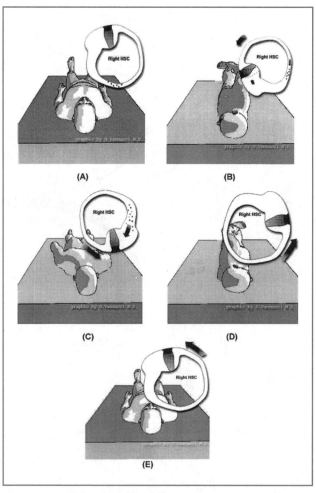

FIGURE 6–28. A–E. The "barbecue" canalith repositioning procedure in a patient with right-sided horizontal semicircular canal (HSC) BPPV. This maneuver is used in cases where the observed nystagmus is geotropic and the canaliths are located in the posterior arm of the horizontal canal. (From Casani et al., 2002)

1. The patient is placed in the supine position.
2. The patient is rotated 90° onto the side of the healthy ear. The patient is held in the position for 90 s starting when the feeling of vertigo has stopped.
3. A second rotation of 90° is made in the same direction placing the patient in the prone position. The patient is held in the position for 90 s starting when the feeling of vertigo has stopped.
4. Another 90° rotation is made in the same direction placing the patient on the side of the impaired ear. The patient is held in the position for 90 s starting when the feeling of vertigo has stopped.
5. The patient finishes the maneuver by making a final 90° rotation when in the supine position. The patient is held in the position for 90 s starting when the feeling of vertigo has stopped.
6. The patient is instructed to sleep in the FPP the night of the CRP.

Liberatory Repositioning Maneuver

The procedure for the liberatory repositioning maneuver (Figure 6–29) (Asprella Libonati et al., 1999) is as follows:

1. The patient is asked to sit on the exam table with his or her legs hanging over the side, his or her upper arms close to the trunk, and his or her hands on their thighs.
2. The patient is rapidly maneuvered toward the healthy side, and the head is quickly rotated 45° downward.
3. The patient is held in this position for at least 90 s starting with when the sensation of vertigo stops.
4. The patient is brought back up into the sitting position.
5. The patient is instructed to sleep in the FPP the night of the CRP.

Apogeotropic HSC-BPPV

Apogeotropic HSC-BPPV is consistently reported as one of the rarest forms of BPPV and has been

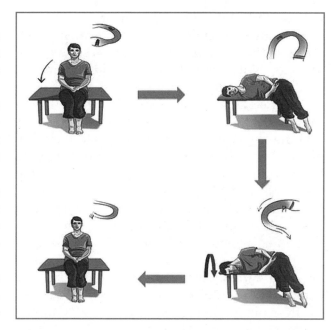

FIGURE 6–29. Illustration of the liberatory maneuver to treat left lateral semicircular canal BPPV when the observed nystagmus is geotropic. (From Casani et al., 2011)

proposed to represent the presence of otolithic debris in the anterior (ampullar) arm near or attached to the cupula. This variant of BPPV generates a bidirectional apogeotropic nystagmus during the supine roll test, the mechanism of which is described earlier in this chapter. Apogeotropic HSC-BPPV has been shown in the literature to be more difficult to treat than geotropic HSC-BPPV (White, Coale, Catalano, & Oas, 2005). This resistance to treatment may be due to the fact that the canaliths are located very close to the ampulla, providing an environment where they can easily adhere to the cupula and create cupulolithiasis. Reports have described three different forms of anterior canal HSC-BPPV. First, the particles can be freely moving in the anterior arm on the canal side of the cupula (see Figure 6–22). In order to treat this form of BPPV, the canaliths must be maneuvered out of the anterior arm into the posterior arm and then into the vestibule. The second variety again involves otolithic matter located on the canal side of the cupula, only the canaliths are attached to the cupula rather than freely moving (cupulolithiasis). In order to treat this form of BPPV, the debris must first be separated from the cupula and then transitioned into the posterior canal and finally the vestibule. The third type involves debris attached to the utricular side of the cupula (see Figure 6–21). In these cases, once the otolithic matter is detached from the cupula, there should be an immediate resolution (the particles migrate directly into the vestibule). Currently, there is no way to differentiate between the two types of cupulolithiasis during the assessment phase.

Once it has been confirmed that the patient has apogeotropic HSC-BPPV, the examiner must determine which of the three variants is causing the symptoms. In an effort to differentiate between canalithiasis and cupulolithiasis, the clinician can perform what has been referred to in the United States literature as the "Gufoni" maneuver (Gufoni, Mastrosimone, & Di Nasso, 1998; Appiani, Catania, Gagliardi, & Cuiuli, 2005). This is a CRP designed to migrate freely moving canaliths from the canal side of the anterior (short) arm of the HSC into the posterior arm (Gufoni et al., 1998; Appiani et al., 2005). This has been termed the "conversion" stage of treatment for apogeotropic HSC-BPPV because the direction of the nystagmus "converts" from apogeotropic to geotropic once the canaliths have been relocated into the posterior arm. There have been several methods described regarding how to accomplish the conversion, yet at the time of this writing no consensus has been reached (Appiani et al., 2005; Casani et al., 2002). The Gufoni maneuver is one such method that has been shown to be successful in transitioning the debris from the anterior arm to the posterior arm of the HSC. Other methods that have been shown to facilitate the treatment of apogeotropic HSC-BPPV include head shaking and FPP (Oh et al., 2009; Vannucchi et al., 1997).

Conversion Technique ("the Gufoni")

The conversion technique, also known as "the Gufoni" (Figure 6–30) (Gufoni et al., 1998), is as follows:

1. The patient is positioned on the side of the exam table facing the examiner.

2. The patient is then briskly maneuvered into a side-lying position on the affected side. The patient is maintained in this position for 120 s starting once the nystagmus is no longer observable.

3. The patient's head is abruptly turned 45° upward and kept in this position for 120 s following the cessation of nystagmus.

4. The patient is returned to the sitting position for 10–15 min.

5. The patient is then positioned supine with the head angled upward 30° so that a supine roll test can be undertaken to determine if the conversion was successful.

Following a conversion maneuver, the clinician can determine if it was successful by repeating the supine head-roll test. If lateral head turns generate a response that is geotropic, the conversion is considered successful and the clinician can perform the traditional HSC-BPPV treatments (e.g., roll CRP or Appiani); however, if the nystagmus continues to be apogeotropic, it can be assumed that the patient has a cupulolithiasis variant and the debris needs to be separated from the cupula (Casani, Giovanni, Bruno, & Luigi, 1997). Several procedures have been described in detail regarding how to detach the otolithic debris from the HSC cupula (Casani et al., 2011; Oh et al., 2009). One such method that has been suggested is head shaking. The patient is laid supine on an exam table with the head elevated approximately 30°. The patient's head is rotated back and forth with approximately 30° arc displacement at a frequency of 2 Hz for 15 s. Following this procedure, a Gufoni maneuver can be performed to move the particles from the anterior arm to the posterior arm, where a supine head-roll test can be performed to determine if the symptoms cease with head turns or if there has been a conversion from apogeotropic to geotropic nystagmus. Another method that has shown to detach the canaliths from the cupula is the FPP (Chiou et al., 2005; Vannucchi et al., 1997). When the FPP is indicated in cases of HSC cupulolithiasis, the patient is instructed to sleep on the side with the weaker response. If a supine head roll assessment is conducted following the FPP, a response manifesting geotropic nystagmus should be produced.

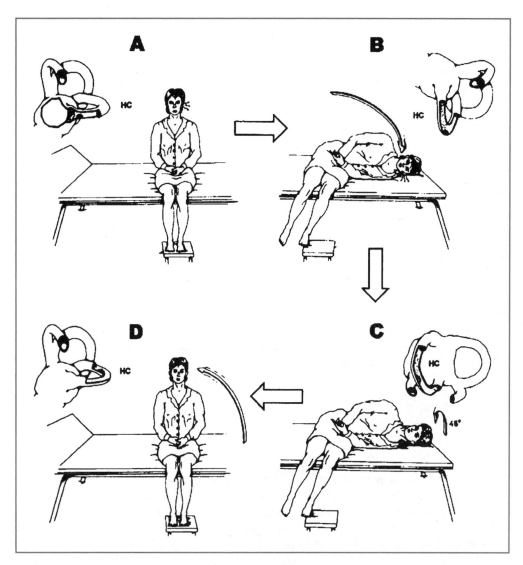

FIGURE 6–30. A–D. A canalith repositioning procedure ("the Gufoni") in a patient with left-sided horizontal semicircular canal BPPV. This maneuver is used in cases where the observed nystagmus is apogeotropic and the canaliths are suspected of being located in the anterior arm of the horizontal canal. This maneuver can be used to convert apogeotropic BPPV into geotropic BPPV. (From Appiani et al., 2005)

Once the canaliths are detached, treatment can be accomplished by performing a liberatory or roll maneuver. Particles that detach from the utricular side of the cupula transition directly into the utricle, resolving the BPPV.

The investigation of how to best treat apogeotropic nystagmus is still developing. While this section provides the background and description of some of the techniques employed, there are numerous other combinations and variations that

have been reported in the literature. Figure 6–31 shows a flow chart that outlines how to use the methods described herein to treat apogeotropic HSC-BPPV.

Treatment of Anterior SCC-BPPV

The treatment of HSC-BPPV and PSC-BPPV is the subject of numerous studies; however, there

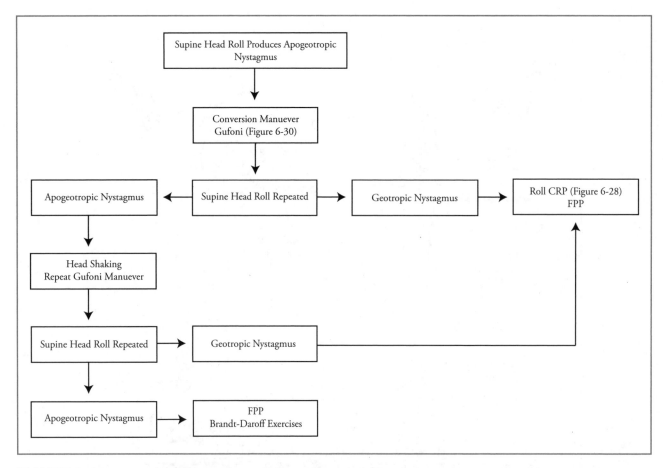

FIGURE 6–31. Algorithm for the treatment of horizontal canal BPPV where the canaliths are located in the anterior portion of the canal (apogeotropic nystagmus observed during the supine roll test). The patient sleeps on the side with the weaker response with the head oriented 45° toward the ground for 12 hr. Head-shaking maneuver: patient's head is moved back and forth 30° in the horizontal plane at a frequency of 2 Hz while the patient is supine with his or her head tilted 30° upward. **FPP** forced prolonged positioning; **CRP** canalith reposition procedure.

is a paucity of data regarding the treatment of ASC-BPPV. One of the first canalith repositioning maneuvers proposed to treat ASC-BPPV was the "reverse Epley" (Honrubia et al., 1999). This procedure consists of using the same method that is employed to treat PSC-BPPV, only the initial head position begins with the head turned toward the unaffected side rather than toward the affected ear. Following the article by Honrubia et al., several other groups of investigators have described additional CRPs to treat ASC-BPPV based on the biomechanical properties (Rahko, 2002; Crevits, 2004). Kim, Shin, and Chung (2005) evaluated and treated 30 patients with ASC-BPPV. The maneuver is based on the concept that freely floating otoconia within the anterior canal should move away from the anterior canal cupula when the head is

rotated away from the affected ear and then lowered at least 30° below the horizontal plane. Kim et al. reported that 96.7% of the patients in this group had complete resolution of their symptoms.

Technique for Treating Anterior Semicircular Canal BPPV

The technique for treating ASC-BPPV (Figure 6–32), based on Kim et al. (2005), is as follows:

1. The patient is seated on a table facing the examiner and the head is turned away from the affected side.
2. A "deep" head-hanging maneuver is performed so that the head is brought to at least

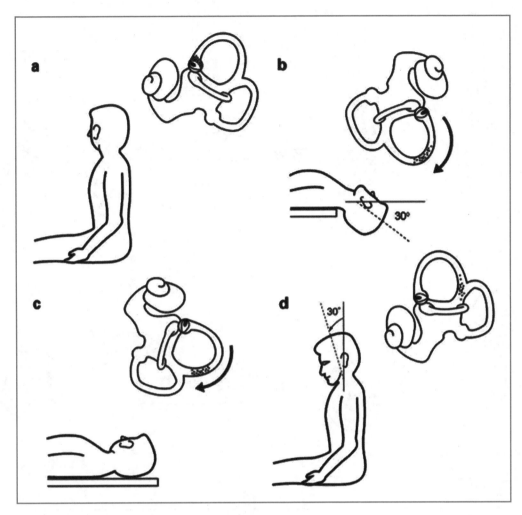

FIGURE 6–32. A–D. A canalith repositioning procedure to treat left anterior semicircular canal BPPV. (From Kim et al., 2005)

30° (preferably 45°) below the horizontal plane for 120 s.

3. The patient's head is lifted into a supine position, keeping the head turned 45° and maintained in the position for 60 s.

4. The patient is brought into the sitting position and the head is moved quickly forward chin to chest.

5. With the chin tilted downward, the patient's head is turned so that it faces forward.

In a certain percentage of patients presenting with ASC-BPPV, the response will be a downbeating nystagmus but with a weak or even absent torsional component (Bertholon et al., 2002). Bertholon et al. suggested that this occurrence is due to the ASC being oriented primarily in the sagittal plane. In cases where there is little or no torsional component, identification of the affected side can be difficult. Yacovino and colleagues (2009) proposed a therapeutic maneuver that is not dependent on identifying the impaired side.

Technique to Treat ASC-BPPV

The technique to treat ASC-BPPV (Figure 6–33), based on Yacovino et al. (2009), is as follows:

1. The patient is seated on a table facing the examiner.

2. A "deep" head-hanging maneuver is performed so that the head is brought to at least 30° (preferably 45°) below the horizontal

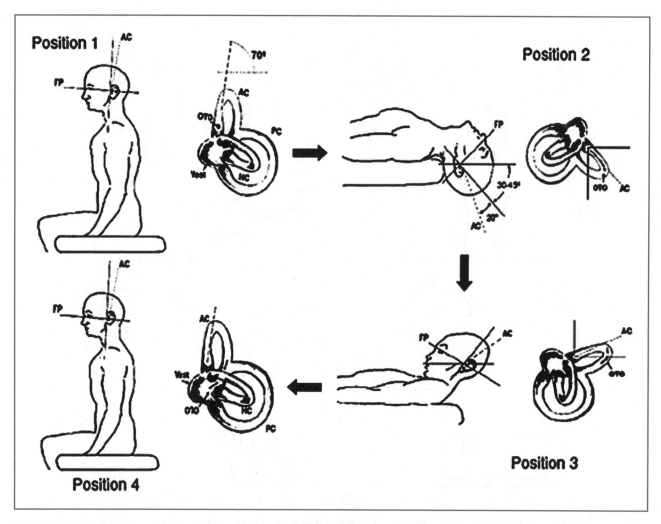

FIGURE 6–33. A canalith repositioning procedure to treat right and left anterior semicircular canal BPPV. **AC** anterior canal; **PC** posterior canal; **HC** horizontal canal; **FP** Frankfort plane. (From Yacovino, Hain, & Gualtieri, 2009)

plane for 2 min. Keep the patient in this position until there is a cessation of the vertigo and nystagmus.

3. The patient's head is lifted into a supine position bringing the chin to the chest.
4. The patient is brought into the sitting position.

Example of Counseling Following the Repositioning Maneuver

Below is an example of counseling following the repositioning maneuver. This form of counseling is used with the counseling material in Appendix B:

Your balance testing was entirely normal with the one exception of the benign paroxysmal position vertigo (BPPV. We found it on one side only and we conducted the particle repositioning maneuver that we felt was appropriate to rid you of this problem. For 2 days try not to do anything that would normally cause you to be dizzy. After 5 days, I would like you to call me at this telephone number and tell me, on a scale of 0–100, what percent better you feel you are on that day compared to this day. Zero percent means that you feel no better on that day than you do today. One hundred percent means that the positional dizziness is completely gone.

Postmaneuver Restrictions

The use of postmaneuver restrictions following the treatment of BPPV has been examined by several groups (Massoud & Ireland, 1996; Roberts et al., 2005). The questions that are asked by investigators typically center on whether there is any benefit in having a patient keep their head in the upright position for 2 or 3 days following a treatment. The evidence appears to be converging on the decision that these post-treatment instructions are unnecessary (Massoud & Ireland, 1996; Nuti, Nati, & Passali, 2000). For example, in a study by Massoud and Ireland (1996), the investigators evaluated the recurrence rate of BPPV in two groups. Both groups were treated with a CRP or liberatory maneuver and asked to sleep upright for two nights and then sleep on the side of the unimpaired ear for five more nights. The second group was treated using the same methods as the first group but were not given any post-treatment instructions. The success rate of the treatment procedures were documented at a follow-up appointment 1 week after the treatment. When the investigators compared the success rates between the two groups, there was no statistical difference. More recently, Nuti et al. (2000) examined the success rate of patients treated for BPPV at different time intervals (i.e., 20 min, 24 hr, and 7 days). Patients were not given any post-maneuver restrictions, and when re-evaluated at 7 days the vast majority of patients were asymptomatic. The conclusion reached by the investigators was that post-maneuver instructions and restrictions are unnecessary.

When Canaliths Repositioning Maneuvers Are Not Successful

Occasionally there are patients who are unable to be maneuvered through a CRP, or after repeated CRPs the BPPV persists. In such instances habituation exercises can be useful. First described by Brandt and Daroff (1980), this treatment for BPPV is able to be performed at home by the patient. The time course for resolution of BPPV using this technique has been reported to take longer than when a conventional CRP is used (Radtke, Neuhauser, von Brevern, & Lempert, 1999).

Brandt-Daroff Exercises for ASC-BPPV and PSC-BPPV

The Brandt-Daroff exercises for ASC-BPPV and PSC-BPPV are as follows:

1. The patient begins by sitting upright and turning his or her head 45° toward the healthy ear.
2. The patient is moved into the side-lying position on the side of the impaired ear keeping the head turned 45°.
3. The patient is kept in the side-lying position until the symptoms of vertigo subside.
4. The patient returns to the original sitting position and remains there for 30 s.
5. The patient turns their head in the opposite direction of step 1 (toward the impaired ear) and moves rapidly into the side-lying position toward the healthy ear.
6. This sequence of exercises is typically recommended to be performed three times (e.g., morning, noon, and night) per day with five repetitions until the vertigo is eliminated.

The Brandt-Daroff exercises can also be modified for BPPV affecting the horizontal SCC. Herdman and Tusa (2007) have described a modified Brandt-Daroff exercise where the same set of procedures as described above is followed. The modification relates to the fact that the head is kept facing forward (not turned 45°) when the patient is moved into the side-lying position. The exact mechanism that results in the Brandt-Daroff exercises resolving the symptoms of BPPV is currently unknown. There are three primary theories regarding how Brandt-Daroff exercises work (Herdman & Tusa, 2007). First, it has been suggested that the movement of endolymph causes the displaced otoconia to eventually dissolve. This may also be why BPPV often remediates without any treatment. Second, the central vestibular nervous system adapts and suppresses the erroneous responses being generated by the peripheral vestibular system. Third, the debris is disconnected from the cupula and moved into a part of the vestibular system where it can no longer generate aberrant responses.

Recurrent BPPV

A certain percentage of patients that are successfully treated for BPPV have a recurrence of the symptoms. Nunez, Cass, and Furman (2000) reported that in their population of patients who reported complete resolution after treatment, there was a recurrence rate of 26.8%. The course of action taken to address the patient with recurrent BPPV depends on a number of patient factors as well the accessibility of the clinician. The ideal method of treatment is to have the patient come back to undergo another assessment and CRP; however, there is a population of patients who continue to present with frequently recurring episodes of BPPV. In these instances it is often disruptive for the patient to have to schedule an appointment for treatment each time a new instance of BPPV arises. Patients who have continually recurring BPPV should be referred to a physician specializing in dizziness. One alternative to having the patient come for treatment with each recurrence is to train the patient to conduct the canalith repositioning maneuver at home (Tanimoto, Doi, Katata, & Nibu, 2005; Radtke et al., 2004; Furman & Hain, 2004).

7

The Caloric Test

INTRODUCTION

The caloric examination is widely considered to be the most technically challenging subtest of the VNG examination but is often the most informative. The primary advantage of caloric testing is the ability to stimulate each labyrinth separately. This ear-specific quantitative information coupled with the caloric tests' high sensitivity to common vestibular impairments continues to make it an important test in the balance clinic. The caloric test consists of two subtests (i.e., measurement of the caloric responses and fixation suppression), each of which evaluates distinctly different processes. If the responses are absent to the caloric irrigations, the ice water caloric test is commonly administered. This chapter describes each component of the caloric test and the role it plays in the VNG/ENG battery.

COMPONENTS OF THE CALORIC TEST

The primary advantage of the caloric test is the information it affords the clinician regarding the physiologic integrity of the right and left horizontal semicircular canals (HSCs) and superior vestibular nerves. The caloric test was originally described by Schmiederkam in the 1860s when he observed that following the irrigation of a patient's ear with water, he could evoke vestibular nystagmus. Barany (1907) is credited with first employing the caloric test to make diagnostic statements regarding the vestibular system. This was later followed by Jung and Mittermaer (1939) describing how to quantify the nystagmus by measuring it via the corneoretinal potential and plotting it for offline analysis. Today's contemporary caloric test consists of two primary components. First, following the irrigation of the external auditory canal with a caloric stimulus, vestibular nystagmus is generated. This peripherally driven response builds to a crescendo and then decays. The examiner typically performs an offline analysis and measures the peak amplitude of the reaction. Second, once the caloric response peaks in amplitude, a measure of vestibulo-ocular (VOR) reflex suppression is taken. Following the "peak" of the caloric response, the fixation-suppression test should be initiated. When a neurologically intact patient is instructed to fixate on a stationary target during the caloric response, the amplitude of the nystagmus attenuates. This phenomenon has been alternately termed "fixation suppression," "VOR suppression," or "VOR cancellation."

Occasionally a patient is encountered where the conventional caloric irrigation does not produce a measurable response from the ear, and it is in these situations that the ice water test is administered (Proctor, 1992). The ice water test is most commonly used to determine if there is any residual function in the ear(s) that did not produce a response during the standard bithermal caloric examination. Ice water approaches a temperature near 10°C while the body maintains a temperature of approximately 37°C (a difference of 27°C) compared with the difference realized by the standard cool caloric irrigation (a difference of 7°C).

INSTRUMENTATION

Caloric Irrigators

At the time of this writing there are two primary types of caloric irrigators available for the caloric test. Each of them has the ability to deliver a calibrated stimulus into the external auditory meatus. The most common irrigator at the moment is the air irrigator followed by the water caloric irrigator. A third less common type of irrigator system known as a closed-loop water system was developed by Kenneth Brookler and Guenter Grams (Figure 7–1). Most irrigators sold today have a thermostat to control and monitor the temperature of the caloric stimulus, a flow meter to control the output of the medium, and a timer. In some instruments the irrigator communicates with a computer that starts and stops the test as well as records the caloric response.

Air Irrigators

While the caloric test has been around since the 1800s, the air irrigator was not commercially available until the mid-1900s (Coats, Herbert, & Atwood, 1976). Most air irrigators are composed of a similar set of components. First, air irrigators typically have an air pump enclosed in the system. Air can also be supplied from a wall source (e.g., larger tertiary medical centers often have these). As the air is pumped through the system it must be heated or cooled. In order to heat the air, Peltier thermoelectric devices are commonly used. These systems run electrical current through a junction between two different metals and thereby heat the air. The amount of heat that is produced depends on the voltage being applied. A thermistor housed in the delivery head samples the temperature of the air and adjusts the voltage to ensure that the air leaving the system is correct. When a cool caloric stimulus is desired, air irrigators often employ radiators. The air is passed through water-filled coils and cooled. Most air irrigators have a small reservoir that holds the water used in this process. The air is typically delivered to the external ear canal using a handset with a tube running through an otoscope specula (Figure 7–2).

While air irrigators are by far the most widely used irrigation systems, they are not without controversy. Numerous reports exist citing the limitations of the caloric responses induced by air (e.g.,

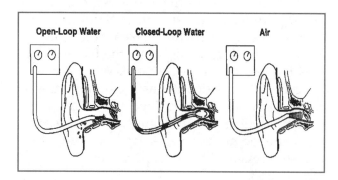

FIGURE 7–1. The three common techniques for caloric irrigation. (From Shepard & Telian, 1996)

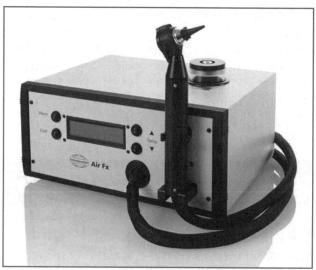

FIGURE 7–2. An example of an air irrigator is shown.

less caloric capacity than water) (Bock & Zangemeister, 1978). For example, the air caloric has been reported to be extremely variable, unreliable, and incapable of generating sufficiently strong responses to measure with any degree of accuracy (Greven, Oosterveld, Rademakers, & Voorhoeve, 1979; Torok, 1979; Zangemeister & Bock, 1980). Reports such as these resulted in the air caloric test not being included in the ANSI standards (ANSI, 1999). Recommendations for the air caloric test were, however, published by the British Standards Association (BSA) in 1999. A recent article by Zapala, Olsholt, and Lundy (2008) suggest that when carefully calibrated, air and water caloric tests elicit similar outcomes. The authors established a method for delivering air irrigations that generated caloric responses equivalent to those produced by water. The recommendations provided by this study and the BSA are presented in Table 7–1 and should be considered when establishing normative data for the caloric test.

Table 7–1. Air Caloric Recommendations

	BSA (1999)	Zapala et al. (2008)
Temperature (°C)	50/24 (±0.4)	51/21
Duration (s)	60 (cool)	60 (warm)/70 (cool)
Volume (L)	8 (±0.5)	8

Water Irrigators

Contemporary water irrigators routinely consist of two reservoirs that store the water for the warm and cool irrigations and a pumping system to deliver the water to the ear. The temperature of the water held in the "baths" is constantly monitored and kept at predetermined irrigation temperatures. Most systems have a foot switch, a hand switch, or both to trigger the transfer of water through the system. The trigger typically consists of a solenoid switch that begins and ends the flow of water based on the settings of a timer. Once the switch is activated, the irrigation is started and the pump begins to move the water from the reservoirs to the head of the delivery system (Figure 7–3). The volume of water being pushed through the system is regulated by a series of valves with settings to increase or decrease the flow rate. It is this elaborate system of valves and tubes that make using distilled water preferable to tap water. Tap water often contains traces of organic material that can accumulate over time and result in costly maintenance fees. Another important point is that many water irrigators monitor and adjust the temperature at the level of the baths and not at the delivery head. The hoses that connect to the delivery head are often insulated in order to maintain the temperature of the water as it travels through the irrigator. An understanding of the workings of the irrigator

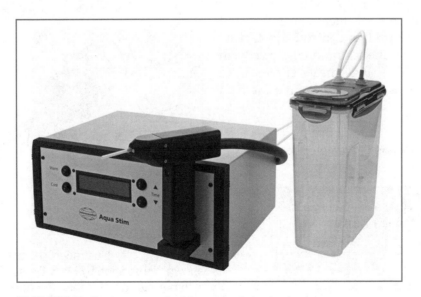

FIGURE 7–3. An example of a water irrigator is shown.

the clinician is using is necessary to avoid pushing standing water that is not the correct temperature into the ear canal. There are some water irrigators that continually circulate the water through the delivery hose. These types of systems ensure that the clinician is ready to irrigate the ear at any point during the exam because the temperature of the water in the hose is continually the same as in the baths. If the irrigator does not continuously circulate the water, it may be necessary to "purge" or run one or two irrigations immediately before administering the caloric stimulus to the patient.

The ANSI and BSA have provided recommended parameters for water irrigations (Table 7–2). Both sets of recommended parameters generate robust caloric responses in the majority of patients, and currently there is no universal agreement on the duration of the stimulus or the flow rate. Each clinic should develop its own normative data or use normative values provided by studies employing similar stimulation techniques.

PREPARATION FOR THE CALORIC TEST

One of the inherent limitations of the caloric test is that the responses are dependent on a multitude of factors, some of which the clinician cannot control. It is the examiner's responsibility to prepare for and address controllable factors (e.g., blocked ear canal) and interpret uncontrollable factors (e.g., tympanic membrane perforation) correctly. In order to accomplish these tasks the tester must have a thorough knowledge of the patient's medical history, a sense of the level of the patient's anxiety, and the current medications that the patient uses.

Inspection of Ear Canals

Prior to caloric testing, the clinician should take a thorough case history. An otoscopic inspection of the ear canal should be performed to identify any anatomic abnormalities (e.g., tympanic membrane perforations or mastoid bowls) for consideration during the analysis and interpretation of the responses. During the otoscopic examination it is not uncommon for the clinician to discover debris in the ear canal. The most common form of debris that is encountered in the external auditory meatus (EAM) is cerumen. Prior to the caloric irrigation, ear wax that significantly occludes the EAM should be removed. A blockage of the ear canal can impede the flow of the irrigation medium and alter the thermal properties of the stimulus being transferred to the lateral semicircular canal. The two most common techniques for removing debris from the EAM are through the use of a curette (Figure 7–4) or water irrigation. The irrigation method of clearing the canal

Table 7–2. Recommended Parameters for Water Irrigations

	BSA (1999)	ANSI (1999)
Temperature (°C)	44/30 (±0.4)	44/30 (±0.5)
Duration (s)	30	40 (±1)
Volume (ml)	250 (±10)	200 (±20)

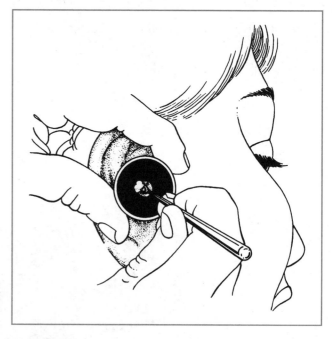

FIGURE 7–4. Illustration of curettage of cerumen is shown. (Illustration by Mary Dersch from Pender, 1992, with permission of Daniel Pender)

is appropriate in cases where a water stimulus is being used to induce the caloric response. Clinics employing air caloric irrigators must be cautious when water is used to clear the ear canal before the caloric test. When warm air is used as the caloric stimulus following a water irrigation, the residual irrigation fluid in the EAM is vaporized. Evaporation is a cooling process, and even though warm air is being delivered into the EAM, the evaporative cooling process produces a decrease in temperature in the EAM. This drop in temperature is radiated through the middle ear space to the vestibule and generates a nystagmus with the fast phase beating toward the non-test ear (Barin, 2008a), opposite the direction that a warm irrigation response normally beats. An otoscopic examination can also provide insight into the size and the shape of the ear canals. Occasionally, patients have extremely tortuous canals that can impede the flow of the air or water through the EAM and produce abnormally reduced caloric responses.

Immediately following the otoscopic examination, the patient should undergo immittance audiometry (tympanograms). The tympanogram provides the examiner with information regarding the status of the middle ear as well as a volume measure of the external ear canal. This can be helpful in confirming that both labyrinths receive equivalent stimulation. In cases where air is being used as the stimulus, a nystagmus that beats in a paradoxical direction can be encountered in patients with tympanic membrane perforations. The mechanism for this is again related to the process of evaporation. When a warm-air stimulus is infused into an ear canal with a tympanic membrane perforation, the warm air enters the middle ear space which has a moist mucosal lining. Once the warm air encounters the wet tissue, evaporative cooling occurs and the temperature in the middle ear space decreases below body temperature. This drop in temperature is transferred to the HSC and creates a caloric response analogous to irrigating with a cool stimulus.

Instructions to Patient

Prior to irrigating the ear, the patient should be informed as to exactly what is going to happen during the caloric test. Patients have a higher tolerance for the procedure if they know what to expect and that any sensation experienced will not last long. It is often helpful to send information to the patient prior to the appointment detailing what tests will be performed and what they involve (Appendix C). In most clinics the caloric test is the last part of the examination, and trust should be established by this point. It is not uncommon for a patient to be apprehensive before the caloric test. If a family member or friend accompanied them to the appointment, it can be helpful to have them stand next to the patient or hold their hand. A thorough case history and scores from the Hospital Anxiety and Depression Scale (HADS) (Zigmond & Snaith, 1983) can be helpful in predicting how a patient will react to either the irrigation or the sensation of motion during the response (Chapter 4). In instances where the patient exhibits a high level of anxiety, the test can be modified accordingly (e.g., more time between irrigations). The following is an example of how the professional sets the expectations for a patient before the caloric examination is initiated:

> What I am trying to measure is what percent stronger one inner ear of balance is compared with the other. The only way we can do that is by changing the temperature of the fluid that is in the inner ear. To do this I am going to run some warm (cool) water in your outer ear for about 25 s. The water will be warmer or cooler than your body temperature. Warming your outer ear will change the temperature of the inner ear fluid by a fraction of a degree. This will make the inner ear fluid move a tiny bit, and that normally happens when you move your head. When you move your head your eyes move. So, for about 1 min, I am going to fool your brain into "thinking" your head is moving when it isn't. That will make your eyes move and that is what I am measuring that will tell me how strong your inner ears of balance are. So you may feel like your head is moving a little bit. If you have that sensation, just know that it is short-lived. It will be important for you to keep your eyes open (for VNG; closed for ENG). I will be asking you some questions and watching your eyes for approximately a minute and a half after the water/air stops.

Procedure for Conducting the Alternating Binaural Bithermal Caloric Test (Water and Air)

Preparation of the Patient

After the patient has been given instructions regarding the caloric test, the eye movement recording system should be calibrated (refer to Chapter 4 for a complete review of calibration). The BSA (1999), Committee on Hearing, Bioacoustics, and Biomechanics (CHABA, 1992), and ANSI (1999) standards all provide the recommendation that for ENG recordings, a recalibration should occur prior to each caloric irrigation; however, while this continual recalibration is necessary for ENG, it is not necessary for VNG. When VNG is employed as the recording technique, an initial calibration should be done prior to any testing. Because the video system tracks the pupils, there should be no need to recalibrate the system unless the goggles have been moved. It is often the case that patients ask to remove the goggles between irrigations or adjust them to increase comfort. In these instances, a recalibration of the VNG system is necessary; however, as discussed in Chapter 4, the recording of eye movements using ENG is more technically challenging because of the dynamic nature of the CRP. Specifically, the calibration procedure must be routinely performed throughout the entire test because the strength of the CRP changes over time and is increased by light (Jacobson & McCaslin, 2004). Several manufacturers of computerized VNG/ENG equipment enable the CRP value to be extracted from the calibration data. This allows the clinician to measure the CRP value and determine if the amplitude is sufficient to generate a clear recording (see Chapter 5 for a detailed explanation). Every effort should be made to ensure that the CRP is stabilized before each caloric is initiated.

The most common caloric test position is with the patient laying supine with their head ventroflexed 30° (see Chapter 3 for an explanation regarding caloric stimulation). This orientation aligns the HSCs in the vertical position where the convection current maximally deflects the HSC cupula. If water is being used as a caloric stimulus, a dental towel can be placed immediately under each ear to avoid getting the patient wet if water spills from the basin, and to give the examiner something upon which to rest the catch basin so that both hands are free. Before the caloric irrigation is delivered, visual fixation must be eliminated. If ENG is being used, the examiner should instruct the patient to close their eyes. ENG can be administered with eyes open if the test room is completely dark or if the patient wears goggles to occlude vision. Having an examination room that is completely devoid of light is rare and a potential risk for the examiner (e.g., falling or tripping). When utilizing VNG as the recording method, vision can be eliminated by placing a cover or shield over the front of the goggles. Any light source that is visible to the patient can be fixated on and thereby reduce the caloric responses. The examiner must also be knowledgeable about how much light can leak into the goggles that are being used.

Precaloric Search for Spontaneous Nystagmus

A search for spontaneous nystagmus (SN) should be performed before the first irrigation is administered and while the patient is in the caloric position (head ventroflexed 30°) (Figure 7–5). The patient's eye movements should be recorded in darkness while undergoing "alerting exercises." If any SN is observed over a 30-s period, its characteristics (e.g., nystagmus velocity and direction) are noted and documented for the final caloric analysis.

CALORIC TEST TECHNIQUE

Caloric Response

Following the precaloric search for SN, the clinician should position themselves at a point where he or she has ready access to the ear canal and it is clearly visible. Prior to beginning the irrigation, another set of instructions should be given and the recording system started. In order to reduce the

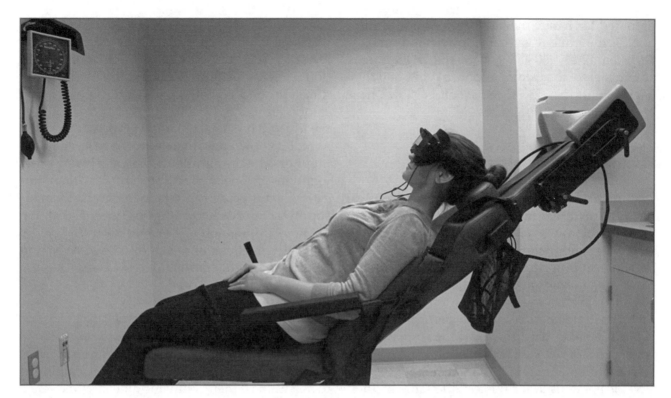

FIGURE 7–5. A patient prepared for caloric testing. Note that the patient is positioned with the head flexed forward approximately 30°.

anxiety of the patient, the examiner should provide an ongoing dialog describing exactly what is happening in the room. Below is an example of an instruction set that could be used immediately before delivering the irrigation:

> I am holding the tube that will run the water (air) into your ear. The water (air) may feel hot, but the ear is sensitive and it should not be painful. I am going to count to three and then the water (air) will begin to run into your ear. Try not to move or jerk your head away when the water (air) enters your ear. The water (air) will run into the ear for 25 s and we will record your eye movements for approximately 2 min afterward. Remember to keep your eyes open (closed if using ENG) and try not to blink too much. I am going to ask you some questions during the test and just do your best to answer them. Here we go . . .

If water is being used for stimulation, the irrigation will continue for 25 s (60 s for air). Immedi-

ately following the end of the irrigation, "alerting exercises" should ensue. Tasking consists of a set of questions (e.g., give me a boy's name that starts with "A") that the patient must think about but can answer easily (a sample list is provided in Appendix E). The process of alerting the patient is critical to obtaining valid recordings for analysis. Patients that are not sufficiently alerted may produce caloric responses that are intermittent or are of insufficient amplitude for analysis. In fact, the process of simply focusing on an imaginary target has been shown to significantly reduce VOR responses (Barr, Schultheis, & Robinson, 1976; Jones, Berthoz, & Segal, 1984). While the exact neural mechanism of the "tasking effect" is not completely understood, it is known that cortical structures provide inhibitory input to the vestibular system at the level of the brainstem. When the cortex is challenged with the tasking exercise, the inhibitory control that the cortex maintains over the brainstem reflex is disrupted and the caloric response emerges. The examiner should be prepared to change the task or speed of the questions if the patient is unable to respond quickly. Approximately 60–90 s after the irrigation is administered, the caloric response peaks and then begins to decline (i.e., the slope of the slow phase becomes less steep) (Figure 7–6).

Fixation Suppression

It is important that the fixation-suppression test be administered immediately after the peak caloric response is reached. This requires that the examiner continually monitor the ongoing caloric response in order to identify when the response reaches its maximum intensity. Depending on the system available and the mode of recording, different methods can be used to perform the test. If ENG is being used to record the response, the tester can simply have the patient open their eyes and fixate on a stationary target (Figure 7–7). If VNG is being used for the test, the same method as used for ENG can be used (i.e., lift the cover and fixate). Most contemporary VNG goggles have light sources inside the goggle system that can be activated during the recordings. The patient should fixate on the target for a period of at least 15 s, and the beginning of when the patient

began to fixate on the target and when vision was once again denied should be marked on the recording (Figure 7–8). One must be careful not to do the fixation-suppression test too early. If fixation suppression is initiated during a point in the caloric reaction where the peak response occurs, the test will be subject to misinterpretation. To the author's knowledge, there is not yet a system that monitors the amplitude of the caloric response, identifies the peak, and then informs the clinician when it is appropriate to begin the fixation-suppression test. According to Alpert (1974), the fixation-suppression test should be administered for both directions of nystagmus (e.g., a fixation measure for right warm and left warm).

Ice Water Caloric Examination

When the caloric responses to standard bithermal stimuli are absent, the ice water test is employed to determine if there is any residual low-frequency function in the test ear(s). The ice water test is conducted with very cold water (i.e., 10°C). Water this temperature can be obtained by placing sterile ice in a cup and then filling it with water (Figure 7–9).

To ensure patient cooperation the test should be explained in detail prior to the irrigation. The

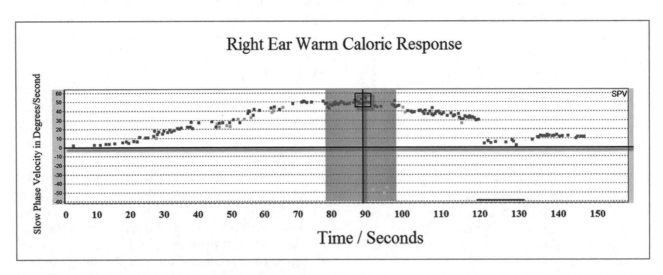

FIGURE 7–6. An example of a slow-phase-velocity profile of a warm caloric response delivered to the right ear. The *dots* represent the measured amplitude (in degrees per second) of the slow phase of each beat of nystagmus. The *box* indicates the peak of the caloric response.

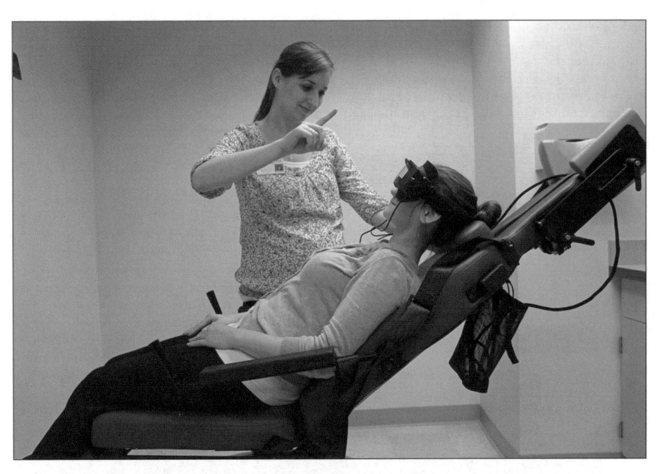

FIGURE 7–7. The fixation suppression test. The patient is asked to orient her gaze on the examiner's finger. This test is initiated immediately following the peak of the caloric response.

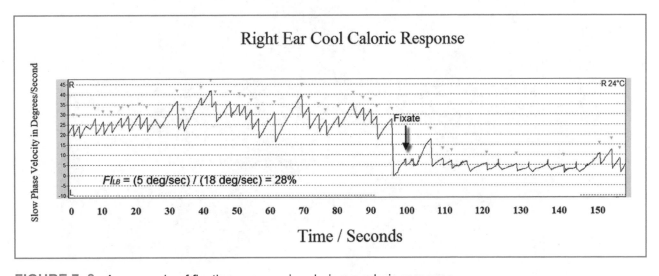

FIGURE 7–8. An example of fixation suppression during a caloric response.

patient should be placed in the standard caloric position and then instructed to turn his or her head so that the test ear is facing upward. A 2-cc syringe can be used to draw water out of the basin. The examiner should then pull the pinna up and back to straighten the ear canal and then gen-

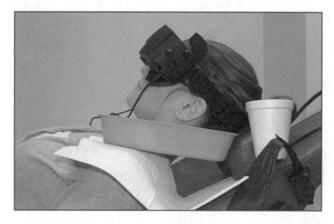

FIGURE 7–9. A patient prepared for the ice water test is shown.

tly fill the ear canal with the water (Figure 7–10). After 20 s, the head should be turned so that the water runs out of the ear canal. The patient should then be provided alerting tasks and the eye movements recorded for at least 60 s. If nystagmus is recorded following the irrigation, and SN has been identified previously that beats in the same direction as the caloric response, the clinician needs to determine whether the response is the SN or a caloric-induced response. This can be accomplished by having the patient change from a supine (face up) to a prone position (face down) with the head hanging downward 30° (Figure 7–11). Each of these positions effectively places the lateral semicircular canals in a position that is parallel to the gravity vector. If the test ear has residual function, that is, if the observed response (nystagmus) is a reaction to the caloric irrigation, it should reverse direction. A change in the direction of the response with a change in the position of the patient suggests that the irrigated ear has some degree of function.

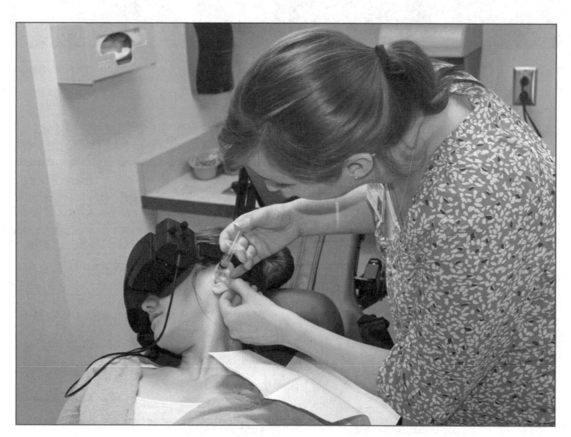

FIGURE 7–10. A patient being irrigated with 2 cc of ice water is shown.

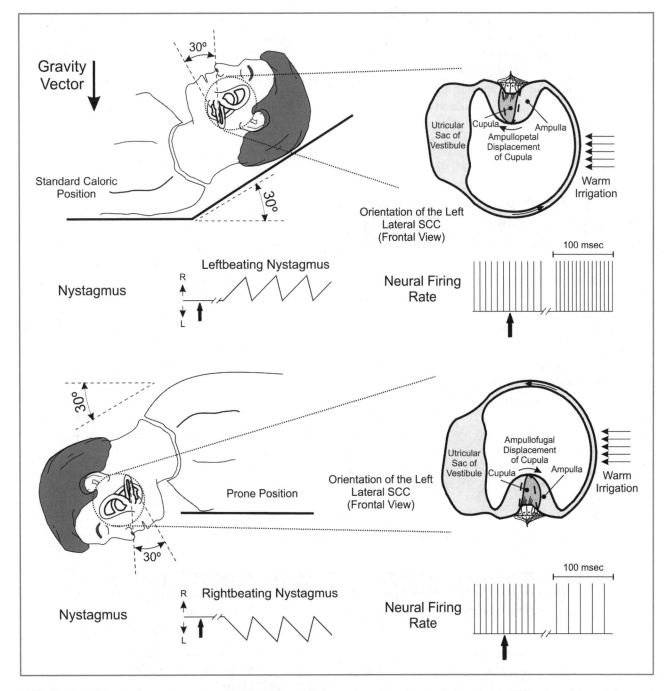

FIGURE 7–11. **A** and **B.** Caloric response in two different head positions. **A.** Supine with the head flexed forward 30° (primary caloric position). **B.** Prone with the head hanging downward 30°. (From Barin, 2009)

Procedure

The procedure for the ice water caloric examination is as follows:

1. Irrigate the ear using ice water (i.e., 10°C)

2. After 20 s, turn the patient's head and drain the water out of the ear canal. The patient's head should be in the primary caloric position.

3. Record the patient's eye movements while looking for caloric-induced nystagmus with

vision denied for 40 s. Alerting should be performed for the duration of the recording.

4. Next, move the patient into the prone position (face down) with the head hanging downward 30°. Record the eye movements again with vision denied and mental alerting for another 40 s. Record any change in the nystagmus.

5. The patient should be returned to the primary caloric position.

ANALYSIS OF CALORIC RESPONSES

It has been reported that the velocity of the slow-phase component of nystagmus taken at the peak of the caloric response is the most useful variable to quantify the reaction (ANSI, 1999; Jacobson, Newman, & Peterson, 1993). According to Jacobson et al. (1993), slow-phase velocity (SPV) of the caloric response can be reported as an average of one of the following four techniques:

1. During the peak of the caloric response, the three beats of nystagmus with the greatest SPV

2. An average of the SPV of all the beats of nystagmus collected during a 5-s period

3. An average of the SPV of all the beats of nystagmus collected during a 10-s period

4. Ten beats obtained at the peak of the caloric response (no time interval specified)

The velocity profile of the caloric response has a characteristic shape when the SPV is plotted on the ordinate and time in seconds on the abscissa. Most commercial VNG systems have either a manual or automatic option for identifying and measuring the velocity of each beat of nystagmus. Once the irrigation begins most systems are triggered to start recording. The velocity profile of the caloric response begins to increase in amplitude approximately 20 s following the onset of the irrigation. The response reaches its peak amplitude at approximately 60–90 s and then begins to decline. The envelope of this response reflects the heat entering and leaving the lateral semicircular canal. In most instances the caloric response is immeasurable at 3 min. When interpreting the caloric test, a series of analyses can be performed that can answer several questions regarding the status of the peripheral vestibular system and the associated central connections. The questions related to these analyses are given in Table 7–3.

Most systems for recording nystagmus plot all four caloric responses on the display simultane-

Table 7–3. Measurement Parameters and Questions Regarding the Peripheral Vestibular System

Measurement Parameters	Questions
Unilateral weakness	Are there interaural (left versus right ear) differences in slow-phase velocity nystagmus?
Directional preponderance	Is there a bias in the direction of the responses (e.g., is right-beating nystagmus always larger than left-beating nystagmus)?
Fixation index	Can the central nervous system appropriately exert control over the vestibular nuclei and reduce amplitude of the caloric nystagmus with visual fixation?
Hypofunction	Is the total of all four caloric responses abnormally low?
Hyperfunction	Is the total of all four caloric responses abnormally high?

ously so that each can be compared with the other. The SPV plots of the caloric response have been termed "pods" because of their lenticular shape (Figure 7–12). While many computerized recording systems automatically perform the analysis outlined in this section, it is important for the clinician to understand what the equations are and how they are used. In this section the variables and measurement parameters used to analyze caloric responses are discussed. The following is how each of the caloric responses is represented in the analysis section (Table 7–4).

Calculation of Total Caloric Response

In order to ensure that the final interpretation of the caloric responses is accurate, the clinician must first determine the sum of the total peak SPV of all four irrigations. When the total peak SPV of the four caloric responses (LW, RW, LC, and RC) is extremely low (e.g., below the 95% lower limit for normal patients), the calculations of traditional caloric parameters is not applicable. In other words, when it is determined that the patient demonstrates significantly reduced responses bilaterally, the clinician should not perform any additional analysis (e.g., unilateral weakness or directional preponderance mea-

sures). This is because very small changes in small caloric responses can result in large changes in the traditional symmetry formulas increasing the likelihood of misinterpretation. To calculate the total caloric response, the peak SPV for each caloric response needs to be assigned and then entered into the following equation:

$$\text{Total caloric response} = RW + LW + RC + LC$$

To determine if a bilateral weakness is present, the clinician must have a set criterion. Several studies of minimum caloric strength have been reported with various conclusions. Barber and Stockwell (1980a) suggested that if a patient's total caloric response is <30° per second, a bilateral weakness exists. Jacobson and Newman (1993)

Table 7–4. Caloric Responses

Caloric Response
Left warm (LW)
Right warm (RW)
Left cool (LC)
Right cool (RC)

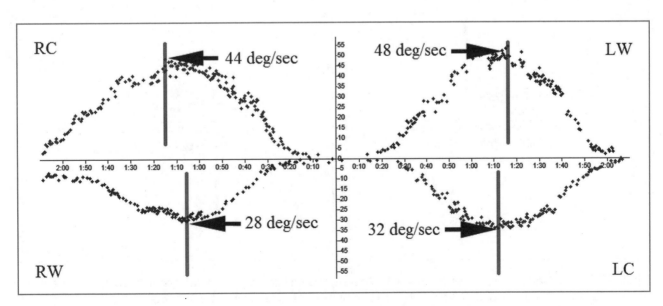

FIGURE 7–12. Caloric responses of a normal patient. **RC** right cool; **RW** right warm; **LW** left warm; **LC** left cool.

have suggested a total caloric response of <22° per second before a patient is considered to have significant bilateral hypofunction. The British Standards Association (1999) operationally defines a bilateral weakness as an examination where each of the four irrigations is <8° per second. Barin (2008a) has suggested incorporating elements from both the Barber and Stockwell (1980a) and Jacobson and Newman (1993) to calculate bilateral weakness. Barin (2008a) requires that the total response for both temperatures from each ear be less than 12° per second (Table 7–5). An example of a patient with a bilateral weakness is presented in Figure 7–13.

Table 7–5. Criteria for Bilateral Weakness

Criterion	Response (degrees/second)
Total right ear peak response (RW + RC)	<12
Total left ear peak response (LW + LC)	<12

Source: From Barin (2008a)

Calculation of Hyperactive Responses

The total caloric response can also be used to determine if the caloric reactions are too large. Caloric responses that exceed the upper limits of normal are classified as hyperactive. The reported criterion varies from maximum SPVs greater than 40° per second to 80° per second. In the classic text by Barber and Stockwell (1980a), a response was qualified as hyperactive if the responses to warm irrigations exceeded 80° per second and cool responses exceeded 50° per second. Jacobson et al. (1993) suggest using the following criterion for defining hyperactive caloric-induced nystagmus (Table 7–6).

Calculation to Determine Symmetry of Function (i.e., Unilateral Weakness)

If the patient does not demonstrate a bilateral weakness, then it is appropriate to continue with further analysis of the caloric responses. The following calculation first proposed by Jongkees and Philipszoon (1964) is designed to compare the difference in caloric responses from the right ear with

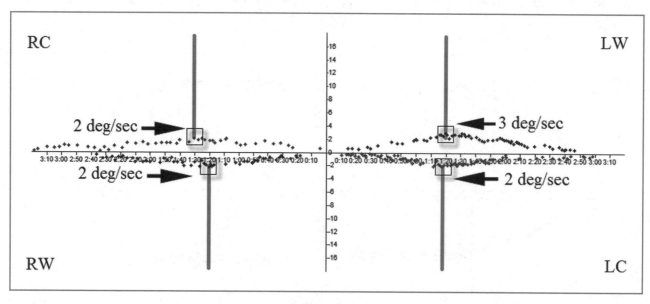

FIGURE 7–13. Caloric responses of a patient with a significant bilateral vestibular system weakness. Total slow-phase velocity = 9° per second. **RC** right cool; **RW** right warm; **LW** left warm; **LC** left cool.

Table 7–6. Criteria for Hyperactive Responses

Criterion	Response (degrees/second)
Total cool peak response (LC + RC)	>99
Total warm peak response (LW + RW)	>146
Total peak response (LC + RC + LW + RW)	>221

Source: From Jacobson et al. (1993)

those from the left ear. The numerator contains the total left ear peak SPV minus the total right ear peak SPV and the denominator is the total peak SPV of all responses summed. This final value is multiplied by 100 to yield a percentage difference. This percentage has been termed a "unilateral weakness" and expresses to what degree the caloric responses from the two ears are different. A positive symmetry value indicates that the left ear is weaker than the right, and a negative number indicates that the right ear is weaker than the left. A unilateral weakness of 100% indicates that there was no measurable caloric response from one of the ears, and a unilateral weakness of 0% indicates that the responses from the two ears were perfectly symmetric (i.e., both ears had the same total SPV for warm and cool caloric responses). When a unilateral weakness is reported it refers to the ear that is weaker (e.g., a right unilateral weakness would be a symmetry measure with a negative number).

The percentage of unilateral weakness is calculated as follows:

$$\text{Unilateral weakness (\%)} = \frac{(LW + LC) - (RW + RC)}{(RC + RW + LC + LW)} \times 100$$

Directional Preponderance

When the standard bithermal caloric test is administered, there are two responses that produce right-beating nystagmus (i.e., right warm and left cool) and two responses that produce left-beating nystagmus (i.e., left warm and right cool). In normal individuals all four of these responses should be approximately equal in amplitude; however, in some instances a patient demonstrates responses that are stronger in one direction than the other. This phenomenon was originally described by Fitzgerald and Hallpike (1942) and is known as a directional preponderance (DP). According to the equation, a positive number is totaled when the caloric responses that produce right-beating nystagmus are stronger than those producing left-beating nystagmus. A negative DP is calculated when the left-beating responses are stronger than right-beating responses, and a value of 0 indicates that they are equal. A DP is conventionally reported in terms of the direction in which the nystagmus is strongest (e.g., if the number is positive, then the patient is reported as having a DP to the right). There are two primary conditions that contribute to the finding of a significant DP. The first, and by far the most common, is the presence of a pre-existing nystagmus that is present with vision denied. The second type is uncommon and has been reported in the literature by Halmagyi et al. (2000) as a "gain asymmetry." Both types of DP must be accounted for in the analysis of the caloric data in order for the clinician to accurately interpret the responses. The equation for calculating the DP percentage is as follows:

$$\text{Directional preponderance (\%)} = \frac{(RW + LC) - (LW + RC)}{(LC + LW + RC + RW)} \times 100$$

Fixation Suppression

The fixation index (FI) is a ratio of nystagmus before and after a patient fixates on a target. Demanez and Ledoux (1970) described this calculation as an assessment of the inhibitory interaction that occurs between the midline cerebellum and the vestibular nuclei. The FI should be calculated once for each direction of nystagmus generated by the caloric response (e.g., right warm and left warm). The process for analyzing the FI consists of the following steps:

1. Identify a 5-s time period just before fixation occurs.
2. Identify a 5-s period after fixation ends.
3. Identify and measure three beats of representative nystagmus in each of the 5-s time periods. If there is no visible nystagmus, its intensity should be qualified 0.
4. Calculate the FI percentage.

The FI percentage is calculated as follows:

$$FI\ (\%) = \frac{SPV\ eyes\ open}{SPV\ eyes\ closed} \times 100$$

Monothermal Warm Caloric Screening Test

The Jongkees and Philipszoon (1964) equation can be adapted to provide a symmetry measure for two warm caloric responses called the monothermal warm screening test (MWST). This screening test of caloric function not only reduces the amount of time required for testing but also can be useful in cases where a patient is unable to continue the test after two irrigations. While the use of two cool irrigations has been reported on as a potential screening measure, it is beyond the scope of this book to discuss them. The MWST was first described by Barber and colleagues (1971), and its performance as a screening measure has since been described in various ways by a number of different groups (Jacobson & Means, 1985; Enticott, Dowell, & O'Leary, 2003; Jacobson, Calder, Shepherd, Rupp, & Newman, 1995; Murnane, Akin, Lynn, & Cyr, 2009). The MWST has been shown to demonstrate a high sensitivity and high specificity for predicting the outcome of the bithermal test if a simple set of rules are followed. Jacobson and Means (1985) presented a set of criteria for when it is appropriate to use the MWST (Table 7–7).

Monothermal warm is calculated as follows:

$$Monothermal\ warm = \frac{RW - LW}{RW + LW} \times 100$$

Table 7–7. Criteria for When to Perform the Monothermal Warm Caloric Screening Test (MWST)

No abnormalities identified during any subtests leading up to the caloric examination.

A MWST can be performed only if each of the warm irrigations exceeds 11° per second.

It is understood that an alternate binaural bithermal caloric examination is performed if the difference between sides exceeds the critical upper limits (i.e., 25% for Jacobson and Means [1985] or 10% for Murnane et al. [2009]).

The fixation suppression test is performed during each warm caloric response.

INTERPRETATION OF CALORIC RESPONSES

Unilateral Weakness

In the author's clinic a significant unilateral weakness is operationally defined as an interaural difference in peak SPV of >22% (Vanderbilt normative data criterion). A significant right unilateral weakness is illustrated in Figure 7–14. The physiologic mechanism of a unilateral weakness stems from an asymmetry in the neural input entering the two vestibular nuclei from the peripheral vestibular system following caloric stimulation. The asymmetry in neural drive to the VOR sets up a situation where the intensity of the caloric-induced nystagmus is larger from the intact side and smaller from the impaired side. Once the responses exceed a difference of greater than 22%, they fall outside the criterion of normal (two standard deviations from a normal mean caloric response) and a patient can be said to have significant peripheral vestibular system impairment. In the case of the caloric examination, "peripheral" refers to structures distal to the vestibular nuclei. This includes the lateral semicircular canal, the superior portion of the vestibular nerve, and the root entry zone of the superior vestibular nerve. In most instances, when a unilateral weakness is identified it can be tracked back to an impairment in one or more of these structures;

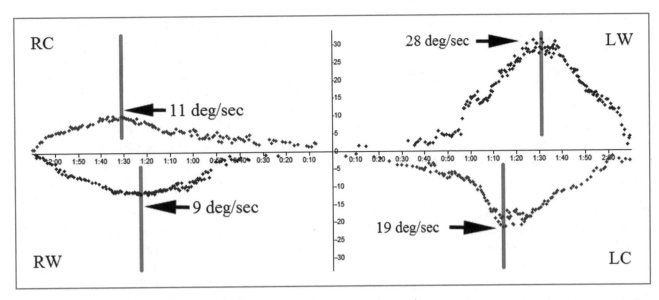

FIGURE 7–14. Caloric responses of a patient with a significant unilateral vestibular system impairment on the right side. **RC** right cool; **RW** right warm; **LW** left warm; **LC** left cool.

however, while the caloric test provides lateralizing information (i.e., it can identify the impaired side), localization between the lateral semicircular canal, superior portion of the eighth cranial nerve, and root entry zone is not possible.

Calculation of caloric weakness for the responses illustrated in Figure 7–14:

$$\text{Unilateral weakness (\%)} =$$

$$\frac{(28 + 19) - (9 + 11)}{(11 + 9 + 19 + 28)} \times 100$$

$$= 40\% \text{ right caloric weakness}$$

According to Stockwell (1990) a unilateral weakness without significant spontaneous nystagmus (>6° per second) is the most common abnormality encountered during VNG testing. These patients often present with symptoms such as the following:

1. Quick head movements that create disorientation
2. Complaints of drifting one way or the other when walking and bumping into people walking next to them
3. A clear event of severe vertigo that may have initiated a visit to the emergency room
4. Hearing loss and ringing in one ear

Once the alternate binaural bithermal test is completed and the unilateral weakness is identified, the examiner should confirm that it is a "true weakness" and not due to some technical error or artifact. During the interpretation of the responses the clinician must be confident that the patient was appropriately alerted during each of the caloric tests and that the irrigations were equivalent. Issues related to confirming that the caloric responses are valid are briefly covered in the "Technical Tips for Caloric Testing" section of this chapter. Once any artifacts or examiner errors have been ruled out, it is safe to document that the patient has unilateral vestibular system impairment on the weak side.

Summary: Unilateral Weakness Abnormalities

The criterion for unilateral weakness abnormalities is >22% asymmetry between the right- and left-side maximum slow-component velocity (based on Vanderbilt normative data). The location of impairment is the unilateral labyrinth, superior portion of the superior vestibular nerve, or root entry zone. It is important to rule out as the cause improper irrigations, lack of alertness, and medications.

Interpretation of Directional Preponderance

The clinical utility of the DP has been debated because of the initial article containing the equation by Jongkees and Phillipzoon (1964). To date, there are two commonly accepted variants of DP (Barin, 2008a). The first variant is observed in patients with a significant degree of SN and is by far the more common. The second type of DP was detailed in a report by Halmagyi, Cremer, Anderson, Murofushi, and Curthoys (2000) and occurs in the absence of SN. The authors have termed this type of DP as "gain asymmetry." The following two sections describe how each type of DP should be approached during analysis and the necessary measures that should be taken to account for it in the final interpretation.

Directional Preponderance in the Presence of Spontaneous Nystagmus

When a unilateral weakness is identified along with significant SN, the analysis becomes more challenging. Spontaneous nystagmus with the slow phase beating toward the side with the impairment is often a sign that the impairment is acute. The very presence of SN implies that compensation mechanisms have not yet equilibrated the neural activity arriving at the vestibular nuclei (one peripheral system is producing more neural input than the other and aberrantly driving the VOR). Patients who have incurred a loss of peripheral vestibular function typically complain of vertigo and/or severe unsteadiness. What is important to account for when interpreting caloric test results from a patient with SN is the effect that the SN has on the peak amplitude of the caloric reaction. Given that peripherally generated SN is direction fixed, caloric responses that generate nystagmus beating in the same direction as the SN are larger (response sums with the SN) than those responses beating in the direction opposite the SN (Fitzgerald & Hallpike, 1942). If the SN is of sufficient amplitude, a significant DP is observed. In the pretest section of this chapter, the technique for searching for pre-existing nystagmus is described. If a significant SN (>6° per second) is identified prior to the caloric examination, it needs to be accounted for during the analysis of the caloric responses. In other words, the examiner must document the amplitude of the SPV of the SN and correct for it in order to provide a true representation of the status of the patient's peripheral vestibular function. The effect of SN on the caloric profile can be described in terms of what happens relative to the recording "baseline." In most instances (not all), a patient with no SN will have a "baseline" near 0. When a caloric stimulus is administered to a patient with no SN, a response emerges at approximately 20 s causing a shift in the baseline activity (either up or down). A patient with a pre-existing SN does not have a starting baseline of 0. Because nystagmus (spontaneous) is present prior to the stimulus being delivered, the system registers this response and the starting baseline is shifted up or down relative to the direction and amplitude of the SN. This concept is illustrated in Figure 7–15.

Calculation of the directional preponderance for the responses illustrated in Figure 7–15:

$$\text{DP (\%)} = \frac{(\text{Total RB}) - (\text{Total LB})}{(\text{Total RB}) + (\text{Total LB})}$$

$$= \frac{(0) - (38)}{(0 + 38)} \times 100 = 100\% \text{ DP to the left}$$

SN should always be accounted for in the final analysis of the caloric responses. Traditionally, the influence of SN on caloric is corrected for by adding or subtracting it from the peak response of the reactions. When SN is identified, its amplitude (in degrees per second) should be calculated by measuring five representative beats over a 20-s period and averaging them. Once the velocity of the SN is calculated, it must be either subtracted or added to each caloric response. The reason for this is that a right-beating SN sums with the response generated by a right warm caloric (right-beating nystagmus) and subtracts from a right cool (left-beating nystagmus). In this way the SN biases the caloric responses with nystagmus that beats in the same direction. The corrections presented in Table 7–8 can be performed to address the influence of SN and normalize the caloric results. It is noteworthy that some commercially available systems allow the tester to move the baseline up or down during

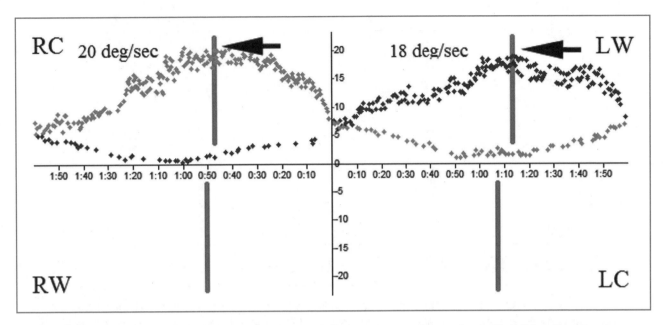

FIGURE 7–15. An example of a significant directional preponderance in a patient with left-beating spontaneous nystagmus. Note that the baseline is shifted 7° to the left (i.e., expressed with respect to the direction of spontaneous nystagmus fast phases). **Peak SPV** peak slow phase velocity; **RC** right cool; **RW** right warm; **LW** left warm; **LC** left cool.

Table 7–8. Correction for Directional Preponderance for Direction-Fixed Spontaneous Nystagmus (*SN*)

Direction of SN	Caloric Response	Correction
Right-beating SN (degrees/second)	Peak right warm (RW)	RW − SN degrees/second = CPR
	Peak left warm (LW)	LW + SN degrees/second = CPR
	Peak right cool (RC)	RC + SN degrees/second = CPR
	Peak left cool (LC)	LC − SN degrees/second = CPR
Left-beating SN (degrees/second)	Peak right warm (RW)	RW + SN degrees/second = CPR
	Peak left warm (LW)	LW − SN degrees/second = CPR
	Peak right cool (RC)	RC − SN degrees/second = CPR
	Peak left cool (LC)	LC + SN degrees/second = CPR

CPR = corrected peak response

Note. Once the caloric responses have been corrected for, the SN for the corrected values should be entered into the formula for calculating unilateral weakness and recalculated.

the analysis portion of the caloric profile in order to account for SN (Figure 7–16).

Calculation of the directional preponderance for the baseline adjusted (7° to the left) responses illustrated in Figure 7–16:

$$DP\ (\%) = \frac{(\text{Total RB}) - (\text{Total LB})}{(\text{Total RB}) + (\text{Total LB})}$$

$$= \frac{(14 - 24)}{(14 + 24)} \times 100 = 26\% \text{ DP to the left}$$

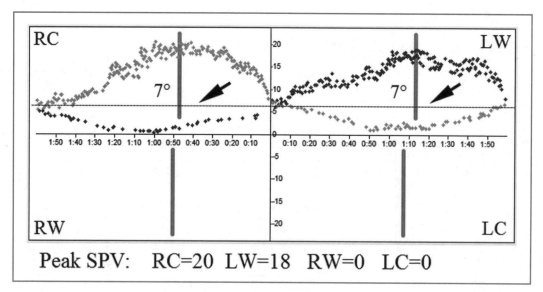

FIGURE 7–16. An example of how the baseline can be moved (*arrows*) to adjust for the spontaneous nystagmus. Baseline average is shifted 7° to the left (corrected for in the accompanying equation). Note how the value of the directional preponderance is reduced following this adjustment. **RC** right cool; **RW** right warm; **LW** left warm; **LC** left cool.

Correction for Directional Preponderance When There Is a Gain Asymmetry

A DP resulting from a gain asymmetry creates a dilemma in the final analysis of the caloric data (Figure 7–17). This is because there is no pre-existing SN value to subtract or add to the caloric responses. In order to correct the caloric responses in cases of gain asymmetry, an examination of the baseline from each of the caloric responses should be recorded. This can be done by measuring the nystagmus in the first 10–15 s of the recording (Barin, 2008a). A baseline average (BL$_{avg}$) can then be calculated using a fraction where the numerator is the sum of the baseline values from each caloric response divided by total number of caloric response administered (i.e., 4). This BL$_{avg}$ value effectively controls for the effect of gain asymmetry and allows the clinician to accurately interpret the caloric response without any central influence.

It is noteworthy that the following formula for calculating gain asymmetry can also be applied to cases where the baseline has been shifted due to the presence of SN (Barin, 2008a). Procedure to correct for a directional preponderance in the presence of a gain asymmetry:

Step 1—Calculate the average baseline asymmetry (BL$_{avg}$):

$$AVG_{BL} = \frac{(RW_{BL} + LW_{BL} + RC_{BL} + LC_{BL})}{4}$$

Step 2—Correct (subtract) AVG$_{BL}$ from each caloric response (Table 7–9).

Step 3—Once the caloric responses have been corrected for, the corrected peak responses should be entered into the gain asymmetry formula (Barin & Stockwell, 2002).

$$\text{Gain Asymmetry (\%)} = \frac{CPR\ RB - CPR\ LB}{CPR\ RB + CPR\ LB} \times 100$$

Summary: Significance of a Directional Preponderance

The criterion for a DP is >28% asymmetry between the left-beating and right-beating maximum SPV (based on Vanderbilt normative data). The mechanisms of impairment are interaction of caloric-induced nystagmus with SN and enhanced dynamic gain of the vestibular nucleus on the impaired side. It is conventional to report baseline shift in the direction of the higher intensity slow phase. In contrast, a gain asymmetry is reported in the direction of the higher intensity fast phases. To avoid misidentifying the cause of DP, it is important to rule out improper irrigations.

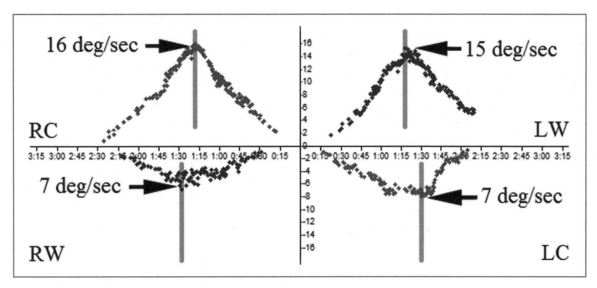

FIGURE 7–17. An example of a directional preponderance with significant gain asymmetry (*arrows*). Note that the baseline is approximately 0. **RC** right cool; **RW** right warm; **LW** left warm; **LC** left cool.

Table 7–9. Correction for Directional Preponderance When There Is a Gain Asymmetry

Baseline Average (AVG$_{BL}$)	Caloric Response	Correction
Gain Asymmetry	Peak right warm (RW)	RW – AVG$_{BL}$ = CPR
	Peak left warm (LW)	LW – AVG$_{BL}$ = CPR
	Peak right cool (RC)	RC – AVG$_{BL}$ = CPR
	Peak left cool (LC)	LC – AVG$_{BL}$ = CPR
Adjustment for Baseline Shift		
CPR RB = –RW CPR – LC CPR		
CPR LB = RC CPR + LW CPR		

CPR = corrected peak response

Interpretation of VOR Fixation Suppression

The percentage that the VOR is attenuated during the caloric response that is considered normal varies in the literature (Coats, Herbert, & Atwood, 1976). In the author's clinic, patients are considered to have normal fixation suppression if they are able to suppress the caloric response by at least 60% with visual fixation. The neural structures underlying VOR fixation suppression are fairly well described. Fixation suppression has been reported to be largely governed by the cerebellar flocculus, which is a structure known to regulate the VOR. Takemori and Cohen (1974) reported that localized lesions in the flocculus of animals results in impairments in fixation suppression; however, the cerebellum does not appear to be the only contributor to fixation suppression. It has also been reported that there is a strong relationship between fixation suppression and the smooth pursuit system (see Chapter 1 for a review of smooth pursuit). Halmagyi and Gresty (1979), among others, have reported that individuals manifesting impaired fixation suppression commonly have impaired smooth pursuit performance (Alpert, 1974; Kato, Kimura, Aoyagi, Mizukoshi, & Kawasaki, 1977). Because of the diffuse nature of the fixation-suppression circuit, the exact pathways and structures driving fixation suppression are currently unknown. In fact, it has been suggested by Tomlinson and Robinson (1981) that a separate system known as "vestibular cancellation" exists to override vestibular input and reduces nystagmus intensity when required. The gaze-holding system, smooth pursuit system, and the fixation-suppression systems all interact, and often when impairments are seen in one they are observed in the others. Consequently, it is not uncommon for patients with impaired VOR fixation suppression to have impaired pursuit or gaze-evoked nystagmus. An example of impaired VOR fixation during the caloric examination is displayed in Figure 7–18.

Summary: Fixation-Suppression Abnormalities

The criteria for fixation-suppression abnormalities are as follows:

1. VOR fixation suppression is abnormal if it does not attenuate the caloric nystagmus by at least 60% (i.e., a fixation index of 40%) (based on Vanderbilt upper limits).
2. Fixation index
   a. 0% = complete suppression of the caloric nystagmus.
   b. 1–100% = partial suppression of the caloric nystagmus.
   c. >100% = an enhancement in the caloric nystagmus.

Impairment in VOR fixation suppression implicates the neural substrate governing the visual–vestibular interaction (e.g., pursuit system and gaze-holding network). The inferior olives as well as the cerebellar flocculus and/or fiber connections between the vestibular nuclei and the flocculus must be intact to suppress the VOR. In the presence of impaired VOR fixation suppression there are often accompanying oculomotor signs of brainstem and/or cerebellar disease (e.g., impaired saccades, down-beating nystagmus, saccadic pursuit). Unilaterally impaired VOR fixation suppression suggests that the lesion is focal (e.g., vascular or tumor). To avoid misidentifying the causes of fixation-suppression abnormalities, it is important to rule out medications (some can impair the cerebellum).

Ice Water Caloric Test

The ice water caloric test is routinely reserved for situations where the ABBT test produces no measurable caloric response(s) or if caloric testing must be performed at the bedside. Interpretation of the ice water test can be complex when SN is present. In cases where the ice water test is being employed to determine if there is any residual function in a severe unilateral weakness, the examiner must have a good measure of any SN in the supine position. This is because SN typically beats in the direction of the healthy ear. When a cold stimulus is infused into the impaired ear, if there is any residual function the caloric nystag-

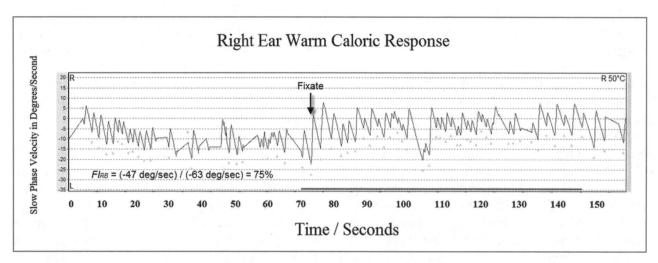

FIGURE 7–18. An example of abnormal fixation suppression during a caloric response.

mus beats toward the healthy ear (in the same direction as the SN); thus, the challenge for the clinician is to determine whether any change in the ongoing nystagmus is due to the caloric response or something else (e.g., alerting). As described in the technique section of the ice water test, the mechanism for elucidating the change in the characteristics of the SN is from the caloric stimulation or from placing the patient in the prone position. Figure 7–19 illustrates the nystagmus profile for a patient with SN who had a positive response when he was transitioned from the supine to the prone position. Table 7–10 illustrates the process of interpreting the ice water caloric test.

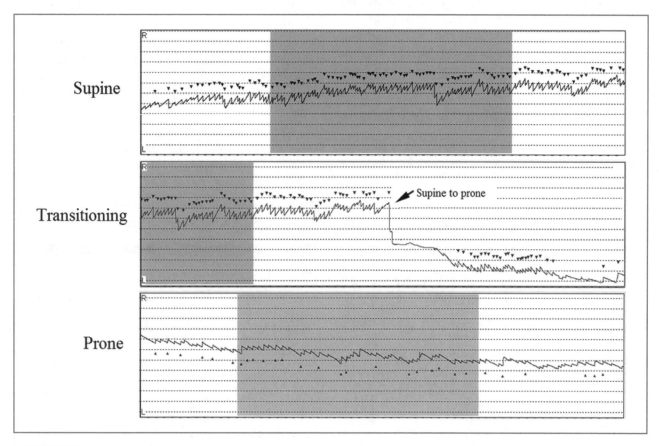

FIGURE 7–19. Caloric responses in a patient following an ice water irrigation of the right ear. The patient has a left-beating spontaneous nystagmus in the supine position that changes to right-beating nystagmus upon transitioning to the prone position.

Table 7–10. Position and Response Following an Ice Water Irrigation of the Right Ear

Supine	Prone/Sitting, Head Tilted	Interpretation
Left-beating nystagmus	Right-beating nystagmus	Positive canal response
Left-beating nystagmus	No nystagmus	Positive canal response
Left-beating nystagmus	Left-beating nystagmus	Negative canal response
Right-beating nystagmus	Any condition	Negative canal response
No nystagmus	Any condition	Negative canal response

Source: Adapted from Proctor (1992)

Summary: Bilaterally Hypoactive Caloric Responses

The criterion for bilaterally hypoactive caloric responses is less than 12° per second total SPV for both the right and left ears (each ear must demonstrate at least 12° per second for warm and cool irrigations). The location of impairment is the labyrinth, superior portion of the vestibular nerve, or root entry zone. To avoid misidentifying the cause, it is important to rule out improper irrigations, middle ear pathology, medications, and saccadic defect.

Interpretation of Hyperactive Responses

There is a substantial body of literature reporting the characteristics of hyperactive caloric responses and their origin. The majority of the work converges on the role of the inhibitory connections between the cerebellum and the vestibular nuclei (Dow, 1938). Specifically, when the situation requires, the cerebellum (i.e., nodulus) can inhibit the VOR (Fernández, Alzate, & Lindsay, 1960; Fredrickson & Fernández, 1964). In cases where a patient has an impairment of the nodulus, the inhibitory influence over the vestibular centers is diminished and the vestibular nuclei assume a higher level of activity. Figures 7–20 and 7–21 illustrate the caloric responses and magnetic resonance imaging in a patient with "hyperactive" caloric responses. Examiners who encounter patients with hyperactive responses must interpret them with caution, as factors other than central nervous system disease have been reported to produce abnormally large caloric responses.

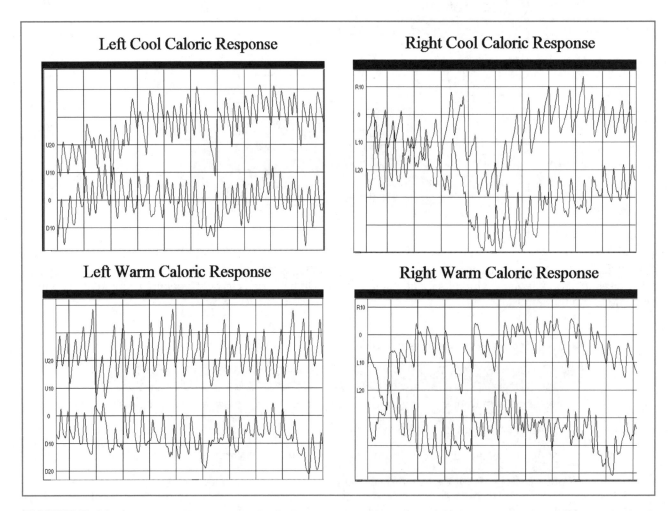

FIGURE 7–20. Example of "hyperactive" caloric responses. Note the vertical nystagmus in addition to the horizontal nystagmus.

For instance, patients who have undergone a mastoidectomy or are extremely anxious can produce larger responses (Figure 7–22). Nonorganic and psychological factors must be accounted for before qualifying a patient as having a cerebellar impairment.

Summary: Hyperactive Responses

The criteria for hyperactive responses are as follows:

1. Total cool peak response (LC + RC) is >99° per second.

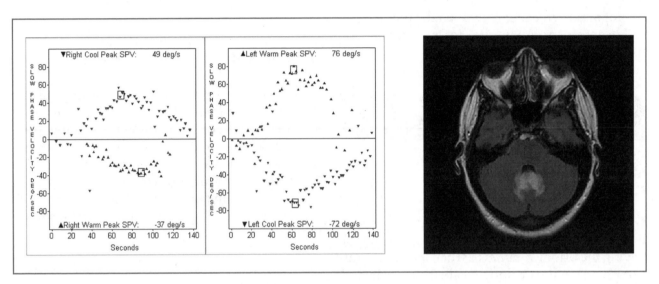

FIGURE 7–21. Caloric pods and a magnetic resonance image with increased enhancement in the midline posterior to the fourth ventricle. Surgical pathology showed this to represent a cerebellar glioma.

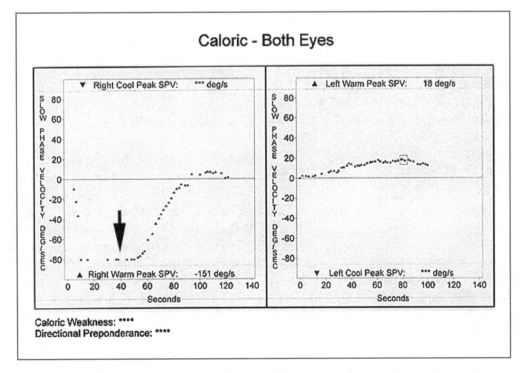

FIGURE 7–22. An example of a caloric response from an ear with a mastoidectomy.

2. Total warm peak response (LW + RW) is >146° per second.
3. Total peak response (LC + RC + LW + RW) is >221° per second.

The location of impairment is the cerebellum (flocculonodular lobe). There is: (a) decreased inhibitory influence on the vestibular nucleus, (b) impaired cerebellar control on the pontine saccade center, and (c) control for nonorganic and psychological contributions.

TECHNICAL TIPS FOR CALORIC TESTING

Interstimulus Interval for Caloric Irrigations

With regard to the interstimulus interval for caloric irrigations, the next caloric should begin 5 min following the prior irrigation or when the nystagmus from the previous caloric has been abolished. A test to determine if there is any residual nystagmus (vision denied with tasking) should always be performed in the caloric position prior to initiating the next caloric.

Order of Irrigations

With regard to the order of irrigations, the author suggests beginning with a warm irrigation in the patient with a normal exam up to the point of caloric testing (allowing for monothermal analysis). Second, irrigate with one temperature and then the other (e.g., RW–LW–RC–LC). Third, if the patient has significant hearing loss, irrigate the ear with the poorer hearing first.

Drugs

With regard to drugs, make sure that the medications that the patient is currently taking are documented in the report and that their effect on the caloric response is accounted for (see Chapter 4 for medication effects).

Abnormal Hyperactive Responses and VOR fixation

Caution should be exercised when interpreting VOR fixation during a hyperactive response. The SPV may be so high that the patient may have a difficult time finding and focusing on the target.

When One Caloric Response Is Significantly Stronger or Weaker

When one caloric response is significantly weaker than the other three, it is typically the result of a poor irrigation or inadequate tasking (Figure 7–23A). When one caloric response is significantly stronger than the other three, it is often the first irrigation performed. This has been suggested to be a result of hyperalertness (Figure 7–23B). The process for resolving the invalid caloric response is as follows:

1. Repeat the outlying irrigation (weakest or strongest).
2. If the repeated response continues to be the same, repeat the other temperature in the same ear as the outlier.
3. If the responses continue to be the same, the patient may need to be brought back for another appointment at a later date. It is not recommended that more than six irrigations be performed consecutively (Barin, 2008a).

Temperature Effect

The temperature effect (Figure 7–24) refers to the effect when one irrigation temperature produces significantly different amplitude responses than the other. This is typically due to poor calibration of the stimulus (e.g., temperature or flow). This effect does not influence the calculations of unilateral weakness or DP and thus in most instances does not change the outcome of the test; however, every effort should be made to have a calibrated system that generates equivalent responses for warm and cool irrigations.

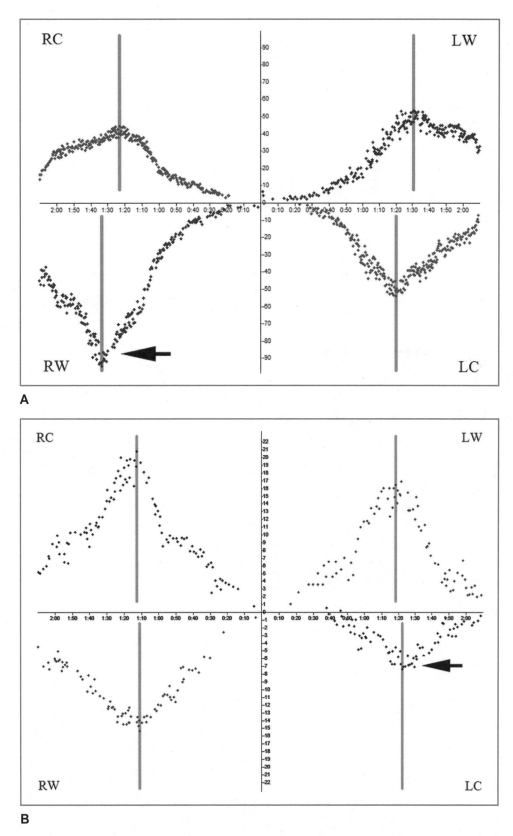

FIGURE 7–23. A and **B.** Two sets of caloric responses that are interpretable and need to be repeated. **A.** A set of caloric responses where one is significantly stronger than the other three. **B.** A set of caloric responses with one response significantly weaker than the other three. The *arrow* indicates the response that is significantly different than the other three. **RC** right cool; **RW** right warm; **LW** left warm; **LC** left cool.

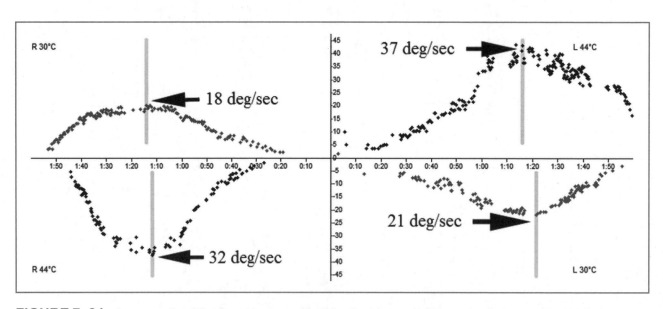

FIGURE 7–24. An example of the "temperature effect" for the binaural bithermal caloric test. Note that the warm responses are significantly stronger than the cool responses.

Appendix

A

Dizziness Questionnaire

Dizziness Questionnaire: Characteristics of Dizziness

IS YOUR DIZZINESSS ASSOCIATED WITH ANY OF THE FOLLOWING SENSATIONS? PLEASE READ THE ENTIRE LIST FIRST. THEN CIRCLE YES OR NO TO DESCRIBE YOUR FEELINGS MOST ACCURATELY.

Yes No   1. Lightheadedness or swimming sensation in the head.

Yes No   2. Blacking out or loss of consciousness.

Yes No   3. Tendency to fall.

Yes No   4. Objects spinning or turning around you.

Yes No   5. Sensation that you are turning or spinning inside, with outside objects remaining stationary.

Yes No   6. Loss of balance when walking in the light: Veering to the Right? Left?

Yes No   7. Loss of balance when walking in the dark: Veering to the Right? Left?

Yes No   8. Headache.

Yes No   9. Nausea.

Yes No 10. Vomiting.

Yes No 11. Pressure in the head.

Yes No 12. Tingling in the fingers or toes.

Yes No 13. Tingling around the mouth.

Dizziness Questionnaire: Associated Ear Symptoms

DO YOU HAVE ANY OF THE FOLLOWING SYMPTOMS? PLEASE CIRCLE YES OR NO AND
CIRCLE THE EAR INVOLVED, IF APPLICABLE.

Yes	No	1. Dizziness. Describe dizziness.				
		_____				
Yes	No	2. Difficulty in hearing?	Both Ears	Right	Left
Yes	No	3. Does your hearing change with dizziness? If so, how?			
		_____				
Yes	No	4. Do you have noise in your ears?	Both Ears	Right	Left
Yes	No	5. Does noise change with dizziness? If so, how?			
		_____				
Yes	No	6. Do you have fullness or stuffiness in your ears?	Both Ears	Right	Left
Yes	No	7. Do you have pain in your ears?	Both Ears	Right	Left
Yes	No	8. Do you have a discharge from your ears?	Both Ears	Right	Left

Dizziness Questionnaire: Associated Neurologic Symptoms

HAVE YOU EXPERIENCED ANY OF THE FOLLOWING SYMPTOMS? PLEASE CIRCLE YES OR NO
AND CIRCLE IF CONSTANT OR IN EPISODES.

Yes	No	1. Double vision	Constant	In Episodes
Yes	No	2. Blurred vision	Constant	In Episodes
Yes	No	3. Blindness	Constant	In Episodes
Yes	No	4. Numbness of the face or extremities	Constant	In Episodes
Yes	No	5. Weakness in the arms or legs	Constant	In Episodes
Yes	No	6. Confusion or loss of consciousness	Constant	In Episodes
Yes	No	7. Difficulty with speech	Constant	In Episodes
Yes	No	8. Difficulty with swallowing	Constant	In Episodes
Yes	No	9. Pain in the neck or shoulders	Constant	In Episodes

Dizziness Questionnaire: Past Medical History, Family History, Social History

Yes   No   1. Did you have a history of earaches or ear infections as a child?

Yes   No   2. Did you ever injure your head? When? _____

Yes   No   3. Were you ever unconscious? When? _____

Yes   No   4. Did you suffer from motion sickness before age 12? _____

Yes   No   5. Have you suffered from motion sickness in the last 10 years? _____

Yes   No   6. Do you now take any medications regularly? What?

_____

Yes   No   7. Have you taken medication in the past for dizziness? Which ones?

_____

_____

Yes   No   8. Do you have a past medical history of: Diabetes? Heart disease?

Yes   No   9. Do you have a family history of: Ear disease? Neurologic disease?
Migraine headache?

Yes   No   10. Do you use tobacco in any form? What kind? _____ How much? _____

Yes   No   11. Does caffeine affect your dizziness? How? _____

_____

Yes   No   12. Does alcohol affect your dizziness? How? _____

_____

Dizziness Questionnaire: Time Course and Aggravating Factors

1. When did your dizziness first occur? _____

2. How often do you become dizzy? _____

3. If dizziness occurs in attacks, how long does an attack last? _____

Yes   No   4. Do you have any warning that dizziness is about to start?

Yes   No   5. Does dizziness occur at any particular time of the day or night?

Yes   No   6. Are you completely free of dizziness between attacks?

Yes   No   7. Does change of position make you dizzy? Which movements?

Yes   No   8. Do you become dizzy when rolling over in bed?   To the right?   To the left?

Yes   No   9. Do you know of any possible cause for your dizziness? What?

_____

Yes   No   10. Do you know of anything that will:

                      a. Stop your dizziness or make it better? _____

                      _____

                      b. Make your dizziness worse? _____

                      _____

Yes   No   11. Do you become dizzy when you bend your head forward?
Yes   No   Backward?

Yes   No   12. Do you become dizzy when you cough?
Yes   No   When you sneeze?
Yes   No   When you have a bowel movement?

            13. Can any of the following make your dizziness worse or start an attack?
Yes   No   Fatigue
Yes   No   Exertion
Yes   No   Hunger
Yes   No   Menstrual period
Yes   No   Stress
Yes   No   Emotional upset
Yes   No   Alcohol

Yes   No   14. Do you have any allergies? What? _____

                      _____

Source: From Furman, Cass, & Whitney (2010)

Appendix

B

A Patient's Guide to Benign Paroxysmal Positional Vertigo (BPPV)

A PATIENT'S GUIDE TO
Benign Paroxysmal Positional Vertigo (BPPV)

BENIGN PAROXYSMAL POSITIONAL VERTIGO

There is a common type of dizziness that affects many patients, and occurs more frequently as we get older. This problem has a long name: **benign paroxysmal positional vertigo**. This problem happens usually on one side only, when calcium carbonate crystals from the part of the inner ear migrate into another part of the inner ear where they don't belong. The typical complaint we hear from patients is that they get violently dizzy when tipping their head back. For example, when screwing in a light bulb overhead or, a patient may tell us they get dizzy when rolling over in bed on the left or right side. The dizziness usually begins with a slight delay (from when a patient places their head in the provoking position) and is quite violent. However, if the you remain in that position, the dizziness will subside within 30 seconds. Understandably most people don't remain in the position that long.

The testing you had today has suggested that you have BPPV on the _____ side.

LEFT   RIGHT

TREATMENT

Treatment for BPPV seldom involves medicine or surgery. This is in large part to our understanding of BPPV. It is a mechanical problem. The conventional treatment for the many forms of BPPV is movement of the head and body through a sequence of positions that are designed to move the crystals out of where the should not be, and into a part of the inner ear of balance where they will dissolve and not cause any immediate problems. Usually, the positional treatment (sometimes referred to as canalith repositioning maneuvers, or, particle repositioning maneuvers or by various names like, Epley or Semont Maneuvers) takes no more than 5 or 6 minutes, is associated with little, if any, discomfort, and will provide you with significant relief of symptoms within 7 days.

AFTER THE PROCEDURE

If you have had a particle repositioning maneuver performed today we will ask you to wait at least 10 minutes after the maneuver before going home to avoid any vertigo that may be encountered by the calcium carbonate crystals repositioning themselves. Also, for the next two nights we will ask you to sleep with your head elevated approximately 45 degrees. We would like for you to avoid doing anything that normally would provoke the dizziness for the next seven days. Finally, we would like for you to call us in one week to tell us what percent you are, or, are not improved (100% means completely cured and 0% means no improvement from when you came in to see us for your test.)

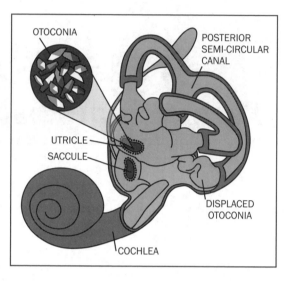

VANDERBILT UNIVERSITY
MEDICAL CENTER

Appendix

C

Vanderbilt Balance Disorders Laboratory Patient Brochure

Vanderbilt Balance Disorders Laboratory

For balance or dizziness-related problems

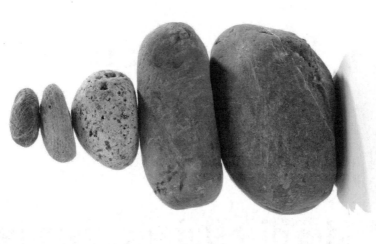

Department of Hearing & Speech Sciences
Division of Audiology
Vanderbilt Bill Wilkerson Center for
Otolaryngology & Communication Sciences

VANDERBILT Ⱳ UNIVERSITY
MEDICAL CENTER

World-class Care

With more than 50 years combined work experience, our staff at the Vanderbilt Balance Disorders Laboratory are experts in balance and dizziness-related problems. We specialize in unique treatment options, and assess conditions using the most current testing techniques and technologies. Our patients receive quality care from specially-trained audiologists who listen, encourage questions and understand your concerns.

VANDERBILT Ⱳ UNIVERSITY
MEDICAL CENTER

Vanderbilt Balance Disorders Laboratory

Vanderbilt Bill Wilkerson Cener
1215 21st Avenue South
Medical Center East, Suite 7209
Phone: 615.343.7084
Fax: 615.322.5833

Vanderbilt Bill Wilkerson Center at Franklin
919 Murfreesboro Road, Suite 200
Franklin, TN 37064
Phone: 615-875-4327

www.vanderbiltbillwilkersoncenter.com

Vanderbilt Balance Disorders Laboratory

The Balance Disorders Laboratory is a diagnostic clinic where specially-trained audiologists conduct tests, the results of which help physicians determine the cause of dizziness, disequilibrium and vertigo. Together with physical therapists, the Balance Disorders Laboratory also conducts assessments of patients who may be at risk for falling. Through this assessment, these specialists can determine what factors place a patient most at risk for falls and make recommendations to the referring physician for reducing that risk. Our goal is to help keep independent seniors independent.

Symptoms of Balance Disorders

- dizziness that is motion-provoked
- vertigo
- tinnitus (ringing in the ears)
- spinning sensation
- headaches
- blurred vision
- falls
- unsteadiness when walking

Normal and Abnormal Function of the Balance System

Most balance disorders are caused by inner ear abnormalities. The normal inner ear of hearing converts sound into a pattern of electricity that the hearing part of the brain understands as meaningful sound. In that way the inner ear of hearing acts exactly like a microphone. The inner ears of balance change movement of the head into patterns of electricity and make it possible for your brain to accurately sense motion in all directions.

Our evaluation is designed to answer these questions:

- Do you have a weak inner ear on one side or both sides?
- Is it the left or right side that is weak?
- How weak is it (20%? 50%? 100%?)
- If you have lost some function on one side, has your brain successfully re-adjusted itself to accommodate the loss of function?

Balance Assessments

There are many tests that can help find the cause of your balance problem. We answer many of these questions by measuring the movements of your eyes with special computerized eyeglasses.

Electronystagmography/ Videonystagmography:

An Electronystagmography test determines how much weaker or stronger the left inner ear of balance is compared to the right. We will record the movements of your eyes as you follow light patterns. We will pretend you are lying down in order to identify vertigo that is caused by changing position. This problem can often be fixed by a simple exercise. With water, we will try to fool your brain, for a very short period of time, into thinking your head is moving when it is not moving at all.

Rotary Chair Test:

If you have had your hearing tested you know that we are interested in knowing how sensitive your hearing system is to sounds of different pitches. We have the same interest in the inner ears of balance. For this test we will record your eye movements as you sit in a chair that swivels from side to side (in much the same way that you would turn an office chair with your feet). *Only available at our Vanderbilt Medical Center East location.*

Vestibular Evoked Myogenic Potential (VEMP) Test:

A VEMP test evaluates the part of the inner ear of balance that reacts to up and down movements of the body. We record muscle tension in your neck following the presentation of brief, moderately loud tones.

Electrocochleography (ECochG):

We will place a silver thread in your outer ear and then a tiny earphone after it. The earphone will make moderately loud clicking sounds. We will record from your outer ear electrical signals the inner ear produces when it creates the electrical code destined for your brain.

Risk of Falls Assessment

Falls are frightening events that can result in hip injuries, hospitalizations and loss of independence. Our falls risk assessments look at factors and warning signs known to cause future falls. Aside from assessing function of the inner ears of balance, the falls risk assessment includes measures of ten factors including blood-pressure, reaction time, and sensation in the feet, ankles and knees.

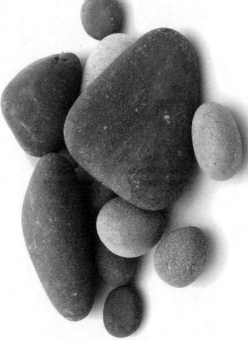

Appendix

D

Your Balance in 4 Pages Counseling Material

YOUR **BALANCE** IN ④ PAGES

WHAT IS THE BALANCE SYSTEM?

You were referred to our clinic because you have spoken with your doctor about your symptoms of dizziness, lightheadedness, or unsteadiness. Dizziness is a term used to broadly describe how we feel when our sense of balance is impaired. Dizziness also is the second most common complaint that patients report to their doctors. The sensations of dizziness are not the same for all people and you should know that there are many medical problems that cause the symptoms that patients report as vertigo, unsteadiness, wooziness, dizziness, and, lightheadedness that are not related to the inner ears of balance. These include circulatory problems, low blood sugar, and, thyroid disorders, just to name a few.

When you report dizziness to your doctor, the challenge is to determine what is causing this sensation.

Diagnosing the underlying cause of a dizziness problem is a complex process often requiring several tests that collectively are referred to as a **balance function assessment**. In addition to the inner ears, we use the senses of vision, and the somatosenses to help maintain our balance and orientation. The somatosenses include touch, pressure, vibration and position senses. Vision tells us where we are with respect to the horizon. The **somatosenses**, for our purposes, refer to our ability to sense vibration, pressure and position of the feet, ankles and knees.

The tests you had today focused on the dizziness or vertigo that can be caused by a disturbance in a particular part of the inner ear called the **vestibular system**. This is the part of your balance system that provides your brain with information about movements of the head and head and body together. The vestibular system informs the brain about movement of the head and body. When the inner ears of balance are not working properly you might receive false senses of movement (you might feel like you are moving when you are not moving at all.) Also, since the inner ear of hearing is physically connected to the inner ear of balance they may both be impaired at the same time. In this situation you may experience hearing loss, and ringing in the ears in addition to dizziness.

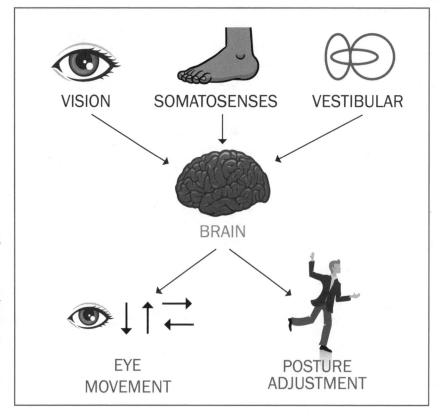

VISION SOMATOSENSES VESTIBULAR

BRAIN

EYE MOVEMENT

POSTURE ADJUSTMENT

HOW DOES MY INNER EAR OF BALANCE WORK?

Instead of having one inner ear of hearing on each side we have five inner ears of balance on each side. Like the inner ears of hearing, the inner ears of balance are filled with fluid and have nerve fibers that are stimulated by movement of your head. The five inner ears of balance on each side make it possible for your brain to know where your head is moving to, and how quickly it is moving.

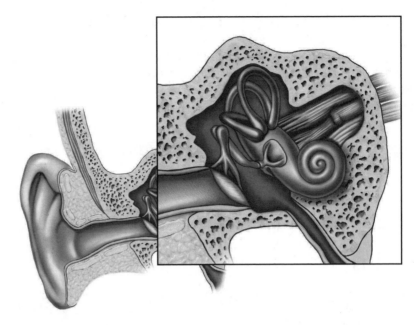

The inner ears of balance are connected with a number of other parts of your brain. For instance, your inner ear of balance connects to brain pathways that move your eyes. In this way, when you turn your head to the right, your eyes automatically move to the left. Alternately, when you turn your head to the left, your eyes automatically move to the right. These are inner ear reflexes. Your inner ears of balance also connect to your spinal cord pathways. It is these connections that make it possible for your brain to detect when you are losing your balance and to correct your posture to keep you from falling over.

The inner ears of balance send electricity to the brain...even when you are sitting still! When you are sitting still, both inner ears of balance send equal amounts of electricity to the brain. It is this equilibrium that your brain interprets as sitting still. When you turn your head to the right, the right inner ear sends more electricity to the brain and the left inner ear sends less (and in darkness an inner ear reflex moves your eyes to the left). When you turn to the left the opposite happens, the left inner ear sends more electricity to the brain and the right inner ear sends less (and in darkness the opposite happens and the inner ear reflex moves your eyes to the right). Now, consider what would happen if you were sitting still but your left inner ear stopped sending electricity to the brain.

In this situation, your brain would be receiving more electricity from the right inner ear, which normally would happen if you were rotating to the right side. In this situation, even though you knew you were sitting still, your brain would be receiving an electrical code it normally would receive if you were turning to the right and that is, indeed, the sensation you would experience.

Also, the eye reflex, in the opposite direction, that normally occurs when you turn your head would make you see things moving in front of you. When patients say they are dizzy we begin to think that possibly they may have a weak inner ear of balance on one side. We will work as a team to figure this out.

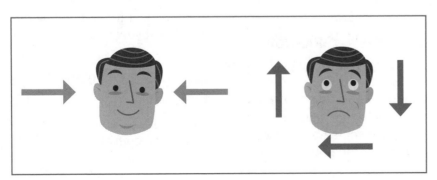

WHAT WERE THE RESULTS OF MY TESTS? DO I HAVE A WEAK INNER EAR?

Today you have undergone a series of tests that are designed to tell us to what degree one inner ear of balance is stronger than the other. The result of these examinations have shown us that your _____ inner ears are weaker than normal.

LEFT	RIGHT	BOTH	NEITHER (you had a normal test)

The caloric examination (water test) has told us that your

LEFT	RIGHT

inner ear is _____% weaker than the other (a difference of 22% or more is considered significant).

WHAT HAPPENS NOW IF I HAVE LOST FUNCTION IN ONE OF MY INNER EARS OF BALANCE?

In most cases, if you lose your hearing in one ear it is permanently gone. If you lose your vision in one eye it is also usually permanently gone. However, if you lose function in one inner ear of balance, your brain, in most cases, has the capability of compensating for this loss so that you are not dizzy forever. In fact, when we lose all, or part, of one inner ear of balance, if we remain safely active, and, if medications that chemically disconnect the inner ear from the brain are not used for long periods of time (these can include vestibular suppressant medications), the brain will compensate for this loss.

Exceptions to this rule are:
1) where brain diseases exist that impede the compensation process,
2) where patients have vestibular diseases that cause the function of the inner ears of balance to change from day-to-day,
3) for elderly patients where the brain connections exist to help compensate, but where they are not as efficient as they were in younger years. In these cases brain compensation may not occur, or, may occur but be less than perfect.

The **rotational test** you had today tells us whether your brain has compensated for a loss of inner ear function on one side.

The results of this test has shown that, if you have a weak inner ear on one side, your brain _____ compensated for the loss of function in your weak inner ear.

HAS	HAS NOT
NOT APPLICABLE	

Another cause of dizziness is having weak or absent function in both inner ears. This can be caused by inner ear or balance nerve diseases, or the use of medications that in addition to helping cure disease, can reduce function in the inner ears of balance (and sometimes hearing). Weak function in both inner ears results in a loss of the ability to keep objects from moving in front of us when we are moving. In these cases the surroundings bobble around in front of us as we move. Patients with two weak inner ears rely more on vision and the somatosenses to help them keep their balance. Because of this, patients with weak or absent function in both inner ears fall when they attempt to stand or walk in darkness.

The results of today's testing has shown that you:

DO	DO NOT

have weak, or absent, inner ear function on both sides.

WHAT IS THE EFFECT OF MY BALANCE PROBLEM ON MY ABILITY TO FUNCTION IN EVERYDAY LIFE?

DIZZINESS HANDICAP INVENTORY SCREENING VERSION (DHI - S)	Yes (4)	Sometimes (2)	No (0)
1E Because of your problem, do you feel depressed?			
2P Does walking down a sidewalk increase your problem?			
3E Because of your problem, is it difficult to concentrate?			
4F Because of your problem, is it difficult for you to walk around your house in the dark?			
5P Does bending over increase your problem?			
6F Because of your problem do you restrict your travel for business or recreation?			
7F Does your problem interfere with your job or household responsibilities?			
8E Because of your problem, are you afraid to leave your home without having someone accompany you?			
9E Because of your problem, have you ever been embarrassed in front of others?			
10F Does your problem significantly restrict your participation in social activities such as going out to dinner, going to movies, dancing or to parties?			
TOTAL SCORE			

The results of your testing suggest that you perceive that your dizziness problem has resulted in a _____ self-report dizziness handicap.

MILD   **MODERATE**   **SEVERE**

NOW THAT I HAVE COMPLETED THIS SERIES OF TESTS, WHAT'S NEXT?

Most likely, you are seeing an ear specialist for problems with dizziness/unsteadiness. Depending on the results of your tests, your doctor may arrive at a diagnosis and treat you, or refer you on for additional testing if they are still searching for an answer. Your doctor will discuss with you further the results of your examination today and what treatment(s) might benefit you.

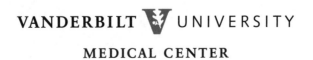

VANDERBILT V **UNIVERSITY**

MEDICAL CENTER

Appendix

E

Example Alerting Tasks for Vestibular Testing

Count . . .

by 3s to 100.

by 4s to 100.

backward by 2s from 100.

backward by 2s from 99.

Name . . .

a woman's name for each letter of the alphabet.

a man's name for each letter of the alphabet.

a city, state, or country for each letter of the alphabet.

an animal for each letter of the alphabet.

something you buy in a grocery store for each letter of the alphabet.

all the U.S. presidents you can recall.

pieces of furniture.

items of clothing.

professional sports or players.

types of flowers or trees.

all the holidays you can recall.

all the colors you can think of.

all the colleges and/or universities.

TV shows/movies (or shows from your childhood).

directions from your house to the _____ clinic.

famous entertainers, musicians, or movie stars.

fruits and/or vegetables.

towns or cities in home state.

For patients that are difficult to task

Name the first names of immediate family and relatives.

Recite a recipe.

Explain what is happening in a television series he or she is watching.

Describe how you would repair a car.

Talk about their hobbies.

Source: From Vanderbilt Balance Disorders Clinic, Nashville, Tennessee

Appendix

F

Reliability and Localizing Value of VNG Findings

Test	Abnormality	Reliability[a]	Localization[b] Peripheral Vestibular	CNS	Comment
Gaze	Horizontal nystagmus (follows Alexander's law)	+++	+++	0	
	Bilateral gaze nystagmus, eyes open	+++	0	+++	
	Bilateral gaze nystagmus, eyes closed	++	0	+++	
	Unilateral gaze nystagmus, eyes open	+++	++	++	
	Unilateral gaze nystagmus, eyes closed	+	0	+	
	Rebound nystagmus	+++	0	+++	Cerebellar system lesion
	Periodic alternating nystagmus	+++	0	+++	Usually posterior fossa lesion
	Up-beating nystagmus	+++	0	+++	Lesion, drug induced
	Down-beating nystagmus	+++	0	+++	Lower medullary lesion
	Pendular nystagmus	+++	0	+++	Usually congenital nystagmus

Test	Abnormality	Reliability[a]	Localization[b] Peripheral Vestibular	CNS	Comment
Gaze *continued*	Square wave movements	++	0	+++	Overalert patient, occasionally cerebellar system lesion
	Internuclear ophthalmoplegia	+++	0	+++	Medial longitudinal fasciculus lesion
Saccade	Ocular dysmetria	+++	0	+++	Cerebellar system lesion
	Saccadic slowing	+++	0	+++	Saccadic system (supranuclear) lesion
	Internuclear ophthalmoplegia	+++	0	+++	Medial longitudinal fasciculus lesion
Tracking	Saccadic pursuit	+++	0	+++	
	Disorganized pursuit	+++	0	+++	
	Disconjugate pursuit	+++	0	+++	
Optokinetic	Asymmetry	+++	0	+++	Supratentorial, brainstem lesion
	Declining response to increasing stimulus speeds	+++	0	+++	Usually brainstem lesion
	Inversion	+++	0	+++	Usually congenital nystagmus
Positional	Direction-fixed nystagmus, eyes open	+++	0	+++	
	Direction-changing nystagmus, eyes open	+++	0	+++	
	Direction-fixed nystagmus, eyes closed	++	++	+	
	Direction-changing nystagmus, eyes closed	++	+	++	If apogeotropic, probably CNS lesion (except PAN II)
	Direction-changing nystagmus, single head position	+++	0	+++	
Dix-Hallpike maneuver	Unilateral benign paroxysmal type positioning nystagmus	+++	++	+	Usually undermost ear lesion
	Bilateral benign paroxysmal type positioning nystagmus	+++	++	++	Both ears, CNS lesion
	All other nystagmus	++	+	++	

Test	Abnormality	Reliability[a]	Localization[b]		Comment
			Peripheral Vestibular	CNS	
Caloric	Unilateral weakness	+++	+++	+	Almost always weak ear lesion
	Directional preponderance	+	+	++	Localization uncertain
	Bilateral weakness	+++	++	+	Both ears, CNS lesion
	Hyperactive response	+	0	+++	Overalert patient, cerebellovestibular disease
	Failure of fixation suppression	+++	0	+++	
	Premature caloric reversal	++	0	+++	
	Caloric inversion	+++	0	+++	Brainstem lesion
	Caloric perversion	+++	0	+++	Brainstem lesion

[a]+++ A "hard" finding, nearly always denotes a lesion; ++ an "intermediate" finding, usually denotes a lesion; + a "soft" finding, sometimes denotes a lesion.

[b]+++ Nearly always denotes the indicated site of lesion; ++ usually denotes the indicated site of lesion; + sometimes denotes the indicated site of lesion; 0 almost never denotes the indicated site of lesion.

Source: From Barber & Stockwell (1980b)

References

Agarwal, Y., Carey, J. P., Della Santina, C. C., Schubert, M. C., & Minor, L. B. (2009). Disorders of balance and vestibular function in US adults: Data from the National Health and Nutrition Examination Survey, 2001–2004. *Archives of Internal Medicine, 169,* 938–944.

Alpert, J. N. (1974). Failure of fixation suppression: A pathologic effect of vision on caloric nystagmus. *Neurology, 24,* 891–896.

American Academy of Otolaryngology-Head and Neck Surgery Committee on Hearing and Equilibrium. (1995). Committee on hearing and equilibrium guidelines for the diagnosis and evaluation of therapy in Meniere's disease. *Otolaryngology-Head and Neck Surgery, 113,* 181–185.

ANSI. (1999). Procedures for testing basic vestibular function. *American National Standards Institute,* BSR S3.45-200, revision of ANSI S3.45.

Appiani, G. C., Catania, G., Gagliardi, M., & Cuiuli, G. (2005). Repositioning maneuver for the treatment of the apogeotropic variant of horizontal canal benign paroxysmal positional vertigo. *Otology & Neurotology, 26,* 257–860.

Asprella Libonati, G. (2005). Diagnostic and treatment strategy of lateral semicircular canal canalolithiasis. *Acta Otolaryngologica Italica, 25,* 277–283.

Baloh, R. W. (1998a). Vertigo. *Lancet, 352,* 1841–1846.

Baloh, R. W. (1998b). *Dizziness, hearing loss, and tinnitus.* Philadelphia, PA: Davis.

Baloh, R. W., & Furman, J. M. (1989). Modern vestibular function testing. *Western Journal of Medicine, 150,* 59–67.

Baloh, R. W., & Honrubia, V. (1990). *Clinical neurophysiology of the vestibular system* (2nd ed.). New York, NY: Oxford University Press.

Baloh, R. W., & Honrubia, V. (2001). *Clinical neurophysiology of the vestibular system* (3rd ed.). New York, NY: Oxford University Press.

Baloh, R. W., Honrubia, V., & Jacobson, K. (1987). Benign positional vertigo: Clinical and oculographic features in 240 cases. *Neurology, 37,* 371–378.

Baloh, R. W., & Kerber, K. A. (2011). *Clinical neurophysiology of the vestibular system* (4th ed.). New York, NY: Oxford University Press.

Baloh, R. W., Konrad, H. R., Dirks, D., & Honrubia, V. (1976). Cerebellar-pontine angle tumors. Results of quantitative vestibulo-ocular testing. *Archives of Neurology, 33,* 507–512.

Baloh, R. W., & Spooner, J. W. (1981). Downbeat nystagmus: a type of central vestibular nystagmus. *Neurology, 31,* 304–310.

Baloh, R. W., Yee, R. D., & Honrubia, V. (1980). Optokinetic nystagmus and parietal lobe lesions. *Annals of Neurology, 7,* 269–276.

Barany, R. (1907). *Physiologie und Pathologie des Bogengangapparates beim Menshen.* Vienna, Austria: Deuticke.

Barber, H. O., & Stockwell C. W. (1976). *Manual of electronystagmography* (1st ed.). St. Louis, MO: Mosby.

Barber, H. O., & Stockwell, C. W. (1980). *Manual of electronystagmography* (2nd ed.). St. Louis, MO: Mosby.

Barber, H. O., & Wright, G. (1973). Positional nystagmus in normals. *Advances in Oto-Rhino-Laryngology, 19,* 276–283.

Barber, H. O., Wright, G., & Demanuele, F. (1971). The hot caloric test as a clinical screening device. *Archives of Otolaryngology, 94*(4), 335–337.

Barin, K. (2008a). Interpretation and usefulness of caloric testing. In G. P. Jacobson & N. T. Shepard (Eds.), *Balance function assessment and management* (pp. 230–252). San Diego, CA: Plural.

Barin, K. (2008b). Interpretation of static position testing in VNG/ENG. In *Insights in Practice for Clinical Audiology,* May, 1–6.

Barin, K. (2009). Neurophysiology of the vestibular system. In J. Katz, L. Medwetsky, & R. Burkhart (Eds.),

Handbook of clinical audiology (6th ed., pp. 431–466). Philadelphia, PA: Lippincott Williams and Wilkinson.

Barin, K., & Durrant, J. D. (2000). Applied physiology of the vestibular system. In R. F. Canalis, & P. R. Lambert (Eds.), *The ear: Comprehensive otology* (pp. 113–140). Philadelphia, PA: Lippincott Williams & Wilkins.

Barin, K., & Stockwell, C. W. (2002). Directional preponderance revisited. In *Insights in practice* (pp. 1–6). Denmark: Otometrics.

Barr, C. C., Schultheis, L. W., & Robinson, D. A. (1976). Voluntary, non-visual control of the human vestibulo-ocular reflex. *Acta Otolaryngolica, 81*, 365–375.

Bennett, M. (2008). The vertigo case history. In G. P. Jacobson & N. T. Shepard (Eds.), *Balance function assessment and management* (pp. 45–62). San Diego, CA: Plural.

Beraneck, M., McKee, J. L., Aleisa, M., & Cullen, K. E. (2008). Asymmetric recovery in cerebellar-deficient mice following unilateral labyrinthectomy. *Journal of Neurophysiology, 100*, 945–958.

Bertholon, P., Bronstein, A. M., Davies, R. A., Rudge, P., & Thilo, K. V. (2002). Positional down beating nystagmus in 50 patients: Cerebellar disorders and possible anterior semicircular canalithiasis. *Journal of Neurology, Neurosurgery & Psychiatry, 72*, 366–372.

Berthoz, A. (1996). How does the cerebral cortex process and utilize vestibular signals? In R. W. Baloh & G. M. Halmagyi (Eds.), *Disorders of the vestibular system* (pp. 113–125). New York, NY: Oxford University Press.

Bhattacharyya, N., Baugh, R. F., Orvidas, L., Barrs, D., Bronston, L. J., Cass, S., . . . & Haidari, J. (2008). Clinical practice guideline: Benign paroxysmal positional vertigo. *Otolaryngology—Head & Neck Surgery, 139*(5 Suppl. 4), S47–S81.

British Society of Audiology (BSA), Balance Interest Group. (1999). Caloric test protocol. *British Journal of Audiology, 33*(3), 179–184.

Bock, O., & Zangemeister, W. H. (1978). A mathematical model of air and water caloric nystagmus. *Biological Cybernetics, 24*, 91–95.

Bojrab, D. I., & McFeely, W. J. (2001). Taking the history: The nature of the spell. In J. A. Goebel (Ed.), *Practical management of the dizzy patient* (pp. 17–22). Philadelphia, PA: Lippincott Williams & Wilkins.

Brandt, T. (1990). Positional and positioning vertigo and nystagmus. *Journal of the Neurological Sciences, 95*, 3–28.

Brandt, T. (1993). Background, technique, interpretation, and usefulness of positional and positioning testing. In G. P. Jacobson, C. W. Newmand, & J. M. Kartush (Eds.), *Handbook of balance function testing* (pp. 123–155). New York, NY: Elsevier.

Brandt, T., & Daroff, R. B. (1980). Physical therapy of benign paroxysmal positional vertigo. *Archives of Otolaryngology, 106*, 484–485.

Bruns, L. (1908). *Geschwulste des Nervensystems.* Berlin, Germany: S. Karger.

Brichta, A. M., & Goldberg, J. M. (1996). Afferent and efferent responses from morphological fiber classes in the turtle posterior crista. *Annals of the New York Academy of Sciences, 78*, 183–195.

Cakir, B. O., Ercan, I., Cakir, Z. A., Civelek, S., Sayin, I., & Turgut, S. (2006). What is the true incidence of horizontal semicircular canal benign paroxysmal positional vertigo? *Otolaryngology—Head & Neck Surgery, 134*, 451–454.

Carl, J. R. (1997). Principles and techniques of electro-oculography. In G. P. Jacobson, C. W. Newman, & J. M. Kartush (Eds.), *Handbook of balance function testing* (pp. 69–82). San Diego, CA: Singular.

Caruso, G., & Nuti, D. (2005). Epidemiological data from 2270 PPV patients. *Audiological Medicine, 3*, 7–11.

Casani, A., Giovanni, V., Bruno, F., & Luigi, G. P. (1997). Positional vertigo and ageotropic bidirectional nystagmus. *Laryngoscope, 107*, 807–813.

Casani, A. P., Nacci, A., Dallan, I., Panicucci, E., Gufoni, M., & Sellari-Franceschini, S. (2011). Horizontal semicircular canal benign paroxysmal positional vertigo: Effectiveness of two different methods of treatment. *Audiology & Neurotology, 16*, 175–184.

Casani, A. P., Vannucci, G., Fattori, B., & Berrettini, S. (2002). The treatment of horizontal canal positional vertigo: Our experience in 66 cases. *Laryngoscope, 112*, 172–178.

Cawthorne, T. (1944). The physiological basis for head exercises. *Chartered Society of Physiotherapy, 30*, 106–107.

Chiou, W. Y., Lee, H. L., Tsai, S. C., Yu, T. H., & Lee X. X. (2005). A single therapy for all subtypes of horizontal canal positional vertigo. *Laryngoscope, 115*, 1432–1435.

Choung, Y. H., Shin, Y. R., Kahng, H., Park, K., & Choi, S. J. (2006). "Bow and lean test" to determine the affected ear of horizontal canal benign paroxysmal positional vertigo. *Laryngoscope, 116*(10), 1776–1781.

Ciuffreda, K. J., Kenyon, R. V., & Stark, L. (1978). Increased saccadic latencies in amblyopic eyes. *Investigative Ophthalmology and Vision Science, 17*, 697–702.

Coats, A. C. (1993). Computer-quantified positional nystagmus in normals. *American Journal of Otolaryngology, 14*, 314–326.

Coats, A. C., Herbert, F., & Atwood, G. R. (1976). The air caloric test. *Archives of Otolaryngology, 102*, 343–354.

Coats, A. C., & Smith, S. Y. (1967). Body position and the intensity of caloric nystagmus. *Acta Otolaryngologica, 63*, 515–532.

Cohen, H. S. (2004). Side-lying as an alternative to the Dix-Hallpike test of the posterior canal. *Otology & Neurotology, 25*, 130–134.

Cohen, H. S., & Jerabek, J. (1999). Efficacy of treatments for posterior canal benign paroxysmal positional vertigo. *Laryngoscope, 109*(4), 584–590.

Cohen, H. S., & Kimball, K. T. (2005). Effectiveness of treatments for benign paroxysmal positional vertigo of the posterior canal. *Otology & Neurotology, 26*, 1034–1040.

Committee on Hearing, Bioacoustics, and Biomechanics (CHABA). (1992). Evaluation of tests for vestibular function. *Aviation, Space, and Environmental Medicine, 63*(2, Suppl.), A1–A34.

Committee on Hearing and Equilibrium guidelines for the diagnosis and evaluation of therapy in Menière's disease. *American Academy of Otolaryngology-Head and Neck Foundation, Inc. Otolaryngology Head and Neck Surgery, 113*, 181–185.

Crevits, L. (2004). Treatment of anterior canal benign paroxysmal positional vertigo by a prolonged forced position procedure. *Journal of Neurology Neurosurgery & Psychiatry, 75*, 779–781.

Croxson, G.R., Moffat, D.A., &Baguley, D. (1988). Bruns bidirectional nystagmus in cerebellopontine angle tumours. *Clinical Otolaryngololgy and Allied Science, 13*(2), 153–157.

Curthoys, I. S. (2002). Generation of the quick phase of horizontal vestibular nystagmus. *Experimental Brain Research, 143*, 397–405.

Curthoys, I. S., & Halmagyi G. M. (1996). How does the brain compensate for vestibular lesions? In R. W. Baloh & G. M. Halmagyi (Eds.), *Disorders of the vestibular system* (pp.145–154). New York, NY: Oxford University Press.

De la Meilleure, G., Dehaene, I., Depondt, M., Damman, W., Crevits, L., & Vanhooren, G. (1996). Benign paroxysmal positional vertigo of the horizontal canal. *Journal of Neurology, Neurosurgery, and Psychiatry, 60*, 68–71.

Demanez, J. P., & Ledoux, A. (1970). Automatic fixation mechanisms and vestibular stimulation. Their study in central pathology with ocular fixation index during caloric tests. *Advances in Oto-Phino-Laryngology, 17*, 90–98.

Dix, M. R., & Hallpike, C. S. (1952). The pathology, symptomology, and diagnosis of certain common disorders of the vestibular system. *Annals of Otology, Rhinology, and Laryngology, 61*, 987–1016.

Dow, R. S. (1938). Effect of lesions in the vestibular part of the cerebellum in primates. *Archives of Neuropsychology, 40*, 500–520.

Drachman, D. A. (1998). A 69-year-old man with chronic dizziness. *Journal of the American Medical Association, 280*, 2111–2118.

Eggers, S. D. Z., & Zee, D. S. (Eds). (2010). Overview of vestibular and balance disorders. In *Vertigo and imbalance: Clinical neurophysiology of the vestibular system* (pp. 3–4). New York, NY: Elsevier.

Enloe, L. J., & Shields, R. K. (1997). Evaluation of health-related quality of life in individuals with vestibular disease using disease-specific and general outcome measures. *Physical Therapy, 77*, 890–903.

Enticott, J. C., Dowell, R. C., & O'Leary, S. J. (2003). A comparison of the monothermal and bithermal caloric tests. *Journal of Vestibular Research, 13*, 113–119.

Epley, J. M. (1992). The canalith repositioning procedure: for treatment of benign paroxysmal positional vertigo. *Otolaryngology—Head & Neck Surgery, 107*, 399–404.

Ewald, R. (1892). *Physiologische Untersuchungen über das Endorgan des Nervous Octavus.* Weisbaden, Germany: Bergmann.

Fernández, C., Alzate, R., & Lindsay, J. R. (1960). Experimental observations on postural nystagmus. II. Lesions of the nodulus. *Annals of Otology, Rhinology, and Laryngology, 69*, 94–114.

Fernández, C., & Goldberg, J. M. (1976). Physiology of peripheral neurons innervating otolith organs of the squirrel monkey. I. Response to static tilts and to long-duration centrifugal force. *Journal of Neurophysiology, 39*, 970–984.

Fettiplace, R., & Fuchs, P. A. (1999). Mechanisms of hair cell tuning. *Annual Review of Physiology, 61*, 809–834.

Fife, T. D. (1998). Recognition and managemnet of horizontal canal benign positional vertigo. *American Journal of of Otology, 19*, 345–351.

Fife, T. D. (2009). Overview of anatomy and physiology of the vestibular system. In S. D. Z. Eggers & D. S. Zee (Eds.), *Vertigo and imbalance, clinical neurophysiology of the vestibular system* (pp. 5–17). New York, NY: Elsevier.

Fitzgerald, G., & Hallpike, C. S. (1942). Studies in human vestibular function. I. Observations of the directional preponderance of caloric nystagmus resulting from cerebral lesions. *Brain, 65*, 115–137.

Fletcher, W. A., & Sharpe, J. A. (1986). Saccadic eye movement dysfunction in Alzheimer's disease. *Annals of Neurology, 20*, 464–471.

Foster, C. A., & Baloh, R. W. (1996). Drug therapy for vertigo. In R. W. Baloh & G. W. Halmagyi (Eds.), *Disorders of the vestibular system* (pp. 541–550). New York, NY: Oxford University Press.

Fredrickson, J. M., & Fernández, C. (1964). Vestibular disorders in fourth ventricle lesions. Experimental studies in the cat. *Archives of Otolaryngology, 80*, 521–540.

Froehling, D. A., Silverstein, M. D., Mohr, D. N., Beatty, C. W., Offord, K. P., & Ballard, D. J. (1991). Benign positional vertigo: Incidence and prognosis in a population-based study in Olmsted County, Minnesota. *Mayo Clinic Proceedings, 66,* 596–601.

Furman, J. M., & Cass, S. P. (1999). Benign paroxysmal positional vertigo. *New England Journal of Medicine, 341,* 1590–1596.

Furman, J. M., Cass, S. P., & Whitney, S. L. (2010). *Vestibular disorders* (3rd ed.). New York, NY: Oxford University Press.

Furman, J. M., & Hain, T. C. (2004). "Do try this at home": Self-treatment of BPPV. *Neurology, 63*(1), 8–9.

Furman, J. M., & Jacob, R. G. (2001). A clinical taxonomy of dizziness and anxiety in the otoneurological setting. *Journal of Anxiety Disorders, 15*(1–2), 9–26.

Furman, J. M., Wall, C., & Pang, D. L. (1990). Vestibular function in periodic alternating nystagmus. *Brain, 113,* 1425–1439.

Gay, A. J., Newman, N. M., Keltner, J. L., & Stroud, M. H. (1974). *Eye movement disorders.* St. Louis, MO: C.V. Mosby.

Glaser, J. S. (1999). *Neuro-ophthalmology* (3rd ed.). Philadelphia, PA: Lippincott Williams & Wilkins.

Goldberg, J. M., & Fernandez, C. (1971a). Physiology of peripheral neurons innervating semicircular canals of the squirrel monkey. I. Resting discharge and response to constant angular accelerations. *Journal of Neurophysiology, 34,* 635–660.

Goldberg, J. M., & Fernandez, C. (1971b). Physiology of peripheral neurons innervating semicircular canals of the squirrel monkey. 3. Variations among units in their discharge properties. *Journal of Neurophysiology, 34,* 676–684.

Goldberg, J. M., Highstein, S. M., Moschovakis, A. K., & Fernandez, C. (1987). Inputs from regularly and irregularly discharging vestibular nerve afferents to secondary neurons in the vestibular nuclei of the squirrel monkey. I. An electrophysiological analysis. *Journal of Neurophysiology, 58,* 700–718.

Greven, A. J., Oosterveld, W. J., Rademakers, W. J., & Voorhoeve, R. (1979). Caloric vestibular test with the use of air. *Annals of Otology, Rhinology and Laryngolology, 88,* 31–35.

Gufoni, M., Mastrosimone, L., & Di Nasso, F. (1998). Repositioning maneuver in benign paroxysmal vertigo of horizontal semicircular canal. *Acta Otorhinolaryngolica Italy, 18,* 363–367.

Hain, T. C. (1992). Oculomotor testing: Interpretation. In G. P. Jacobson, C. W. Newman, & J. M. Kartush (Eds.), *Handbook of balance function testing* (pp. 83–122). St. Louis, MO: Mosby.

Hain, T. C., & Rudisill, H. (2008). Practical anatomy and physiology of the ocular motor system. In G. P. Jacobson & N. T. Shepard (Eds.), *Balance function assessment and management* (pp. 13–26). San Diego, CA: Plural.

Hajioff, D., Barr-Hamilton, R. M., Colledge, N. R., Lewis, S. J., & Wilson, J. A. (2000). Re-evaluation of normative electronystagmography data in healthy ageing. *Clinical Otolaryngology and Allied Sciences, 25,* 249–252.

Halmagyi, G. M., Cremer, P. D., Anderson, J., Murofushi, T., & Curthoys, I. S. (2000). Isolated directional preponderance of caloric nystagmus: I. Clinical significance. *American Journal of Otology, 21,* 559–567.

Halmagyi, G. M., & Gresty, M. A. (1979). Clinical signs of visual-vestibular interaction. *Journal of Neurology Neurosurgery and Psychiatry, 42,* 934–939.

Han, B. I., Oh, H. J., & Kim, J. S. (2006). Nystagmus while recumbent in horizontal canal benign paroxysmal positional vertigo. *Neurology, 66,* 706–710.

Harrington, J. W. (1969). Caloric stimulation of the labyrinth experimental observations. *Laryngoscope, 79,* 777–793.

Heide, W., Kurzidim, K., & Kömpf, D. (1996). Deficits of smooth pursuit eye movements after frontal and parietal lesions. *Brain, 119,* 1951–1969.

Herdman, S. J. (Ed.). (2007). Physical therapy management of benign positional vertigo. *Vestibular rehabilitation* (3rd ed., pp. 45–62). Philadelphia, PA: Davis.

Herdman, S. J., & Tusa, R. J. (1996). Complications of the canalith repositioning procedure. *Archives of Otolaryngology Head Neck Surgery, 122,* 281–286.

Herdman, S. J., & Tusa, R. J. (2007). Assessment and treatment of patients with benign paroxysmal positional vertigo. In Susan J. Herdman (Ed.), *Vestibular rehabilitation* (pp. 451–475). Philadelphia, PA: F. A. Davis Company.

Herdman, S., Tusa, R., & Clendaniel, R. (1994). Eye movment signs in vertical canal benign paroxysmal positional vertigo. In A. Fuchs, T. Brandt, U. Büttner, & D. Zee, (Eds.), *Contemporary Ocular Motor and Vestibular Research: A Tribute to David A. Robinson* (pp. 385–387). Stuttgart, Germany: Georg Thieme-Verlag.

Herdman, S. J., Tusa, R. J., Zee, D. S., Proctor, L. R., & Mattox, D. E. (1993). Single treatment approaches to benign paroxysmal positional vertigo. *Archives of Otolaryngology—Head & Neck Surgery, 119,* 450–454.

Heywood, S., & Churcher, J. (1981). Direction-specific and position-specific effects upon detection of displacements during saccadic eye movements. *Vision Research, 21,* 255–261.

Hilton, M., & Pinder, D. (2004). The Epley (canalith repositioning) maneuver for benign paroxysmal positional vertigo. *Cochrane Database Systematic Review, 2,* CD003162.

Honrubia, V., Baloh, R. W., Harris, M. R., & Jacobson, K. M. (1999). Paroxysmal positional vertigo syndrome. *American Journal of Otology, 20,* 465–470.

Hood, J. D. (1989). Evidence of direct thermal action upon the vestibular receptors in the caloric test. A re-interpretation of the data of Coats and Smith. *Acta Otolaryngology, 107,* 161–165.

Hotson, J. R., & Baloh, R. W. (1998). Acute vestibular syndrome. *New England Journal of Medicine, 339*(10), 680–685.

Hudspeth, A. J. (1982). Extracellular current flow and the site of transduction by vertebrate hair cells. *Journal of Neuroscience, 2,* 1–10.

Hudspeth, A. J., & Corey, D. P. (1977). Sensitivity, polarity, and conductance change in the response of vertebrate hair cells to controlled mechanical stimuli. *Proceedings of the National Academy of Sciences, 74,* 2407–2411.

Humphriss, R. L., Baguley, D. M., Sparkes,V., Peerman, S. E., & Moffat, D. A. (2003). Contraindications to the Dix-Hallpike manoeuvre: A multidisciplinary review. *International Journal of Audiology, 42,* 166–173.

Imai, T., Ito M., Takeda, N., Uno, A., Matsunaga, T., Sekine, K., & Kubo, T. (2005). Natural course of the remission of vertigo in patients with benign paroxysmal positional vertigo. *Neurology, 64,* 920–921.

Isaacson, J. E., & Rubin, A. M. (1999). Otolaryngologic management of dizziness in the older patient. *Clinical Geriatric Medicine, 1,* 179–191.

Ishiyama, G., Finn, M., Lopez, I., Tang, Y., Baloh, R. W., & Ishiyama, A. (2005). Unbiased quantification of Scarpa's ganglion neurons in aminoglycoside ototoxicity. *Journal of Vestibular Research, 15,* 197–202.

Ishiyama, A., Lopez, I., Ishiyama, G., & Tang, Y. (2004). Unbiased quantification of the microdissected human Scarpa's ganglion neurons. *Laryngoscope, 114,* 1496–1499.

Isotalo, E., Pyykkö, I., Juhola, M., & Aalto, H. (1995). Predictable and pseudo random saccades in patients with acoustic neuroma. *Acta Otolaryngolica, 1*(Suppl. 520), 22–24.

Ito, M. (1993). Neurophysiology of the nodulofloccular system. *Revue Neurologique, 149,* 692–697.

Ito, M., Nisimaru, N., & Yamamoto, M. (1977). Specific patterns of neuronal connexions involved in the control of the rabbit's vestibule-ocular reflexes by the cerebellar flocculus. *Journal of Physiology* (London), *265,* 833–854.

Jackson, L., Morgan, B., Fletcher, J., & Krueger, W. (2007). Anterior canal benign paroxysmal positional vertigo: An underappreciateed entity. *Otology and Neurotology, 28,* 218–222.

Jacobson, G. P., & Calder, J. H. (1998). A screening version of the Dizziness Handicap Inventory (DHI-S). *American Journal of Otology, 19*(6), 804–808.

Jacobson, G. P., Calder, J. A., Shepherd, V. A., Rupp, K. A., & Newman, C. W. (1995). Reappraisal of the monothermal warm caloric screening test. *Annals of Otology, Rhinology, and Laryngology, 104,* 942–945.

Jacobson, G. P., & McCaslin, D. L. (2004). Detection of ophthalmic impairments indirectly with electronystagmography. *Journal of the American Academy of Audiology, 15,* 258–263.

Jacobson, G. P., & Means, E. D. (1985). Efficacy of a monothermal warm water caloric screening test. *Annals of Otology, Rhinology and Laryngology, 4* (Part 1), 377–381.

Jacobson, G. P., & Newman, C. W. (1990). The development of the Dizziness Handicap Inventory. *Archives of Otolaryngology—Head & Neck Surgery, 116,* 424–427.

Jacobson, G. P., & Newman, C. W. (1993). Background and technique of caloric testing. In G. P. Jacobson, C. W. Newman, & J. M. Kartush (Eds.), *Handbook of balance function testing* (pp. 157–192). St. Louis, MO: Mosby Year Book.

Jacobson, G. P., Newman, C. W., Hunter, L., & Balzer, G. K. (1991). Balance function test correlates of the Dizziness Handicap Inventory. *Journal of the American Academy of Audiology, 2,* 253–260.

Jacobson, G. P., Newman, C. W., & Peterson, E. L. (1993). Interpretation and usefulness of caloric testing. In G. P. Jacobson, C. W. Newman, & J. M. Kartush (Eds.), *Handbook of balance function testing* (pp.156–192). St. Louis, MO: Mosby Year Book.

Jacobson, G. P., Pearlstein, R., Henderson, J., Calder, J. H., & Rock, J. (1998). Recovery nystagmus revisited. *Journal of the American Academy of Audiology, 9,* 263–271.

Jacobson, G. P., Shepard, N. T., Dundas, J. A., McCaslin, D. L., & Piker, E. P. (2008). In G. P. Jacobson & N. T. Shepard (Eds.), *Balance function assessment and management.* San Diego, CA: Plural.

Jones, G. M., Berthoz, A., & Segal, B. (1984). Adaptive modification of the vestibulo-ocular reflex by mental effort in darkness. *Experimental Brain Research, 56,* 149–153.

Jongkees, L. B., & Philipszoon, A. J. (1964). Electronystagmography. *Acta Otolaryngology* (Suppl. 189), 189–191.

Jung, R., & Mittermaier, R. (1939). Zur objektiven registrierung und analyse verschiedener nystagmusformen: vestibularer, optokinetischer und spontaner nystagmus in ihren wechselbeziehungen. *European Archives of Otorhinolaryngology, 146,* 410–439.

Kandel, E. R., Schwartz, J. H., & Jessell, T. M. (2000). *Principles of neural science* (4th ed.). New York, NY: McGraw-Hill.

Kato, I., Kimura, Y., Aoyagi, M., Mizukoshi, K., & Kawasaki, T. (1977). Visual suppression of caloric nystagmus in normal individuals. *Acta Otolaryngolica, 83,* 245–251.

Kerber, K. A., Meurer, W. J., West, B. T., & Fendrick, A. M. (2008). Dizziness presentations in U.S. emergency departments, 1995–2004. *Academy of Emergency Medince, 15,* 744–750.

Kim, Y. K., Shin, J. E., & Chung, J. W. (2005). The effect of canalith repositioning for anterior semicircular canal canalithiasis. *Journal of Otorhinolaryngology and Related Specialties, 67,* 56–60.

Kinney, S. E., Sandridge, S. A., & Newman, C. W. (1997). Long-term effects of Ménière's disease on hearing and quality of life. *American Journal of Otology, 18,* 67.

Koo, J. W., Moon, I. J., Shim, W. S., Moon, S. Y., & Kim, J. S. (2006). Value of lying-down nystagmus in the lateralization of horizontal semicircular canal benign paroxysmal positional vertigo. *Otology & Neurotology, 27,* 367–371.

Korres, S., & Balatsouras, D. (2004). Diagnostic, pathophysiologic, and therapeutic aspects of benign paroxysmal positional vertigo. *Otolaryngology-Head and Neck Surgery, 131,* 438–444.

Korres, S., Balatsouras, D. G., Kaberos, A., Economou, C., Kandiloros, D., & Ferekidis, E. (2002). Occurrence of semicircular canal involvement in benign paroxysmal positional vertigo. *Otology & Neurotology, 23,* 926–932.

Leigh, R. J., & Zee, D. S. (2006). *The neurology of eye movements* (4th ed.). New York, NY: Oxford University Press.

Lempert, T. (1994). Horizontal benign positional vertigo. *Neurology, 44,* 2213–2214.

Lightfoot, G. R. (2004). The origin of order effects in the results of the bi-thermal caloric test. *International Journal of Audiology, 43,* 276–282.

Lloyd, S. K., Baguley, D. M., Butler, K., Donnelly, N., & Moffat, D. A. (2009). Bruns' nystagmus in patients with vestibular schwannoma. *Otology & Neurotology, 30*(5), 625–628.

Lysakowski, A. (2005). Anatomy of the vestibular end organs and neural pathways. In W. Cummings (Ed.), *Cummings otolaryngology head and neck surgery* (pp. 3089–3114). Philadelphia, PA: Elsevier.

Marmor, M. F., & Zrenner, E. (1993). Standard for clinical electro-oculography. International Society for Electrophysiology of Vision. *Archives of Ophthalmology, 111,* 601–604.

Marti, S., Palla, A., & Straumann, D. (2002). Gravity dependence of ocular drift in patients with cerebellar downbeat nystagmus. *Annals of Neurology, 52,* 712–721.

Massoud, E. A., & Ireland, D. J. (1996). Post-treatment instructions in the nonsurgical management of benign paroxysmal positional vertigo. *Journal of Otolaryngology, 25,* 121–125.

Mazzoni, A. (1969). Internal auditory canal arterial relations at the porus acusticus. *Annals of Otology, Rhinology, & Laryngology, 78,* 797–814.

McAuley, J. R., Dickman, J. D., Mustain, W., & Anand, V. K. (1996). Positional nystagmus in asymptomatic human subjects. *Otolaryngology—Head & Neck Surgery, 114,* 545–553.

McCaslin, D. L., & Jacobson, G. P. (2009). Current role of the videonystagmography examination in the context of the multidimensional balance function test battery. *Seminars in Hearing, 30,* 242–253.

McCaslin, D. L., Jacobson, G. P., Grantham, S. L., Piker, E. G., & Verghese, S. (2011). The influence of unilateral saccular impairment on functional balance performance and self-report dizziness. *Journal of the American Academy of Audiology, 22*(8), 542–549; quiz 560–561.

McKenna, L., Hallam, R. S., & Hinchcliffe, R. (1991). The prevalence of psychological disturbance in neurotology outpatients. *Clinical Otolaryngology and Allied Sciences, 16,* 452–456.

McLaren, J. W., & Hillman, D. E. (1979). Displacement of the semicircular canal cupula during sinusoidal rotation. *Neuroscience, 4,* 2001–2008.

Mizukoshi, K., Watanabe, Y., Shojaku, H., Okubo, J., & Watanabe I. (1988). Epidemiological studies on benign paroxysmal position vertigo in Japan. *Acta Otolaryngolica, 447,* 67–72.

Money, K. E., Bonen, L., Beatty, J. D., Kuehn, L. A., Sokoloff, M., & Weaver, R. S. (1971). Physical properties of fluids and structures of vestibular apparatus of the pigeon. *American Journal of Physiology, 220,* 140–147.

Moon, S. Y., Kim, J. S., Kim, B. K., Kim, J. I., Lee, H., Son, S. I., . . . Lee, W. S. (2006). Clinical characteristics of benign paroxysmal positional vertigo in Korea: A multicenter study. *Journal of Korean Medical Science, 21,* 539–543.

Murnane, O. D., Akin, F. W., Lynn, S. G., & Cyr, D. G. (2009). Monothermal caloric screening test performance: a relative operating characteristic curve analysis. *Ear and Hearing, 30,* 313–329.

Musiek, F. D., Baran, J. A., Shinn, J. B., & Jones, R. O. (2012). *Disorders of the auditory system.* San Diego, CA: Plural.

Nedzelski, J. M. (1983). Cerebellopontine angle tumors: Bilateral flocculus compression as cause of associated oculomotor abnormalities. *Laryngoscope, 93,* 1251–1260.

Nunez, R. A., Cass, S. P., & Furman, J. M. (2000). Short- and long-term outcomes of canalith repositioning for benign paroxysmal positional vertigo. *Otolaryngology—Head & Neck Surgery, 122,* 647–652.

Nuti, D., Agus, G., Barbieri, M. T., & Passali, D. (1998). The management of horizontal-canal paroxysmal positional vertigo. *Acta Otolaryngolica, 118,* 455–460.

Nuti, D., Nati, C., & Passali, D. (2000). Treatment of benign paroxysmal positional vertigo: No need for postmaneuver restrictions. *Otolaryngology—Head & Neck Surgery, 122,* 440–444.

Nuti, D., Vannucchi, P., & Pagnini, P. (1992). Benign paroxysmal vertigo of the horizontal canal: A form of canalithiasis with variable clinical features. *Journal of Vestibular Research, 6,* 173–184.

Odman, M., & Maire, R. (2008). Chronic subjective dizziness. *Acta Otolaryngolica, 128,* 1085–1088.

Oghalai, J. S., Manolidis, S., Barth, J. L., Stewart, M. G., & Jenkins, H. A. (2000). Unrecognized benign paroxysmal positional vertigo in elderly patients. *Otolaryngology—Head & Neck Surgery, 122,* 630–634.

Oh, S. Y., Kim, J. S., Jeong, S. H., Oh, Y. M., Choi, K. D., Kim, B. K., . . . Lee, J. J. (2009). Treatment of apogeotropic benign positional vertigo: Comparison of therapeutic head-shaking and modified Semont maneuver. *Journal of Neurology, 256,* 1330–1336.

Okada, Y., Takahashi, M., Saito, A., & Kanzaki, J. (1991). Electronystagmographic findings in 147 patients with acoustic neuroma. *Acta Otolaryngolica, 487,* 150–156.

Parnes, L. S., Agrawal, S. K., & Atlas, J. (2003). Diagnosis and management of benign paroxysmal positional vertigo (BPPV). *Canadian Medical Association Journal, 169,* 681–693.

Parnes, L. S., & McClure, J. A. (1991). Posterior semicircular canal occlusion in the normal hearing ear. *Otolaryngology—Head & Neck Surgery, 104,* 52–57.

Parnes, L. S., & McClure, J. A. (1992). Free-floating endolymph particles: A new operative finding during posterior semicircular canal occlusion. *Laryngoscope, 102,* 988–992.

Parnes, L. S., & Price-Jones, R. G. (1993). Particle repositioning maneuver for benign paroxysmal positional vertigo. *Annals of Otology, Rhinology, and Laryngology, 102*(5), 325–331.

Pender, J. D. (1992). *Practical otology.* Philadelphia, PA: J.B. Lippincott.

Pierrot-Deseilligny, C., & Milea, D. (2005). Vertical nystagmus: Clinical facts and hypotheses. *Brain, 128,* 1237–1246.

Proctor, L. R. (1992). The ice water caloric test. *The ENG Report Archives* (pp. 69–72). Denmark: ICS Medical.

Radtke, A., Neuhauser, H., von Brevern, M., & Lempert, T. (1999). A modified Epley's procedure for self-treatment of benign paroxysmal positional vertigo. *Neurology, 53,* 1358–1360.

Radtke, A., von Brevern, M., Tiel-Wilck, K., Mainz-Perchalla, A., Neuhauser, H., & Lempert, T. (2004). Self-treatment of benign paroxysmal positional vertigo: Semont maneuver vs Epley procedure. *Neurology, 63,* 150–152.

Rahko, T. (2002). The test and treatment methods of benign paroxysmal positional vertigo and an addition to the management of vertigo due to the superior vestibular canal (BPPV-SC). *Clinical Otolaryngology & Allied Sciences, 27,* 392–395.

Raphan, T., Matsuo, V., & Cohen, B. (1979). Velocity storage in the vestibulo-ocular reflex arc (VOR). *Experimental Brain Research, 35,* 229–248.

Rasmussen, A. T. (1940). Studies of the VIIIth cranial nerve of man. *Laryngoscope, 50,* 67–83.

Roberts, R., & Gans, R. (2008). Background, technique, interpretation, and usefulness of positional/positioning testing. In G. P. Jacobson & N. T. Shepard (Eds.), *Balance function assessment and management* (pp.171–196). San Diego, CA: Plural.

Robinson, D. A. (1964). The mechanics of human saccadic eye movement. *Journal of Physiology, 174,* 245–264.

Ross, M. D., Donovan, K., & Chee O. (1985). Otoconial morphology in space-flown rats. *Physiologist, 28,* 219–220.

Rucker, J. C. (2010) Overview of anatomy and physiology of the ocular motor system. In S. D. Z. Eggers & D. S. Zee (Eds), *Vertigo and Imbalance: Clinical neurophysiology of the vestibular system* (pp. 18–42). New York, NY: Elsevier.

Ruckenstein, M. (2001). Therapeutic efficacy of the Epley canalith repositioning maneuver. *Laryngoscope, 111,* 940–945.

Ruckenstein, M. J., & Staab, J. P. (2009). Chronic subjective dizziness. *Otolaryngology Clinics of North America, 42,* 71–77.

Salvinelli, F., Firrisi, L., Casale, M., Trivelli, M., D'Ascanio, L., Lamanna, F., . . . Costantino, S. (2004). Benign paroxysmal positional vertigo: Diagnosis and treatment. *La Clinica Terapeutica, 155,* 395–400.

Sato, H., Ohkawa, T., Uchino, Y., & Wilson, V. J. (1997). Excitatory connections between neurons of the central cervical nucleus and vestibular neurons in the cat. *Experimental Brain Research, 115,* 381–386.

Scherer, H., Brandt, U., Clarke, A. H., Merbold, U., & Parker, R. (1986). European vestibular experiments on the Spacelab-1 mission: 3. Caloric nystagmus in microgravity. *Experimental Brain Research, 64,* 255–263.

Schor, C. M. (2003). Neural control of eye movements. In P. L. Kaufman, & A. Alm (Eds.), *Adler's physiology of the eye* (10th ed., pp. 830–858). St. Louis, MO: Mosby.

Schuknecht, H. F. (1962). Positional vertigo. Clinical and experimental observations. *Transactions of the American Academy of Ophthalmology and Otolaryngology, 66,* 319–331.

Schuknecht, H. F. (1969). Cupulothiasis. *Archives of Otolaryngology, 90,* 765–778.

Schukneckt, H. F., & Ruby, R. R. (1973). Cupulothiasis. *Advances in Otorhinolaryngology, 20,* 434–443.

Semont, A., Freyss, G., & Vitte, E. (1988). Curing the BPPV with a liberatory maneuver. *Advances in Otorhinolaryngology, 42,* 290–293.

Shepard, N. T., & Schubert, M. (2008). Interpretation and usefulness of ocular motility testing. In G. P. Jacobson & N. T. Shepard (Eds.), *Balance function assessment and management* (pp. 45–62). San Diego, CA: Plural.

Shepard, N. T., & Telian, S. A. (1996). *Practical management of the balance disorder patient.* San Diego, CA: Singular.

Sherrington, C. S. (1947). *The integrative action of the nervous system.* New Haven, CT: Yale University Press.

Sloane, P. D. (1989). Dizziness in primary care. Results from the National Ambulatory Medical Care Survey. *Journal of Family Practice, 29,* 33–38.

Staab, J. P., & Ruckenstein, M. J. (2005). Chronic dizziness and anxiety: Effect of course of illness on treatment outcome. *Archives of Otolaryngology—Head & Neck Surgery, 131,* 675–679.

Staab, J. P., & Ruckenstein, M. J. (2007). Expanding the differential diagnosis of chronic dizziness. *Archives of Otolaryngology—Head & Neck Surgery, 133,* 170–176.

Straka, H., Biesdorf, S., & Dieringer, N. (2000). Spatial distribution of semicircular canal nerve evoked monosynaptic response components in frog vestibular nuclei. *Brain Research, 880,* 70–83.

Strupp, M., Brandt, T., & Steddin, S., (1995). Horizontal canal benign paroxysmal positional vertigo: Reversible ipsilateral caloric hypoexcitability caused by canalolithiasis? *Neurology, 45,* 2072–2076.

Sylvestre, P. A., & Cullen, K. E. (1999). Quantitative analysis of abducens neuron discharge dynamics during saccadic and slow eye movements. *Journal of Neurophysiology, 82,* 2612–2632.

Takemori, S., & Cohen, B. (1974). Loss of visual suppression of vestibular nystagmus after flocculus lesions. *Brain Research, 72,* 213–224.

Tanimoto, H., Doi, K., Katata, K., & Nibu, K. I. (2005). Self-treatment for benign paroxysmal positional vertigo of the posterior semicircular canal. *Neurology, 65,* 1299–1300.

Timmerman, H. (1994). Pharmacotherapy of vertigo: Any news to be expected? *Acta Otolaryngolica, 513,* 28–32.

Tomlinson, R. D., & Robinson, D. A. (1981). Is the vestibule-ocular reflex cancelled by smooth pursuit? In A. Fuchs & W. Becker (Eds.), *Progress in oculomotor research* (pp. 533–539). New York, NY: Elsevier.

Torok N. (1979). Pitfalls in detecting vestibular decruitment with air calorics. *Journal of Otorhinolaryngology & Related Specialties, 4,* 143–146.

Uchino, Y. (2001). Otolith and semicircular canal inputs to single vestibular neurons in cats. *Uchu Seibutsu Kagaku, 15,* 375–381.

Van Der Stappen, A., Wuyts, F. L., & Van De Heyning, P. H. (2000). Computerized electronystagmography: Normative data revisited. *Acta Otolaryngolica, 120,* 724–730.

Vannucchi, P., Giannoni, B., & Pagnini, P. (1997). Treatment of horizontal semicircular canal benign paroxysmal positional vertigo. *Journal of Vestibular Research, 7,* 1–6.

von Brevern, M., Radtke, A., Lezius, F., Feldmann, M., Ziese, T., Lempert, T., & Neuhauser, H. (2007). Epidemiology of benign paroxysmal positional vertigo: a population based study. *Journal of Neurology, Neurosurgery, and Psychiatry, 78,* 710–715.

von Brevern, M., Schmidt, T., Schönfeld, U., Lempert, T., & Clarke, A. H. (2006) Utricular dysfunction in patients with benign paroxysmal positional vertigo. *Otology & Neurotology, 27,* 92–96.

White, J. A., Coale, K. D., Catalano, P. J., & Oas J. G. (2005). Diagnosis and management of lateral semicircular canal benign paroxysmal positional vertigo, *Otolaryngology—Head & Neck Surgery, 133,* 278–284.

Whitney, S. L., Marchetti, G. F., & Morris, L. O. (2005). Usefulness of the dizziness handicap inventory in the screening for benign paroxysmal positional vertigo. *Otology & Neurotology, 26,* 1027–1033.

Wolf, J., Boyev, K., Manokey, B., & Mattox, D. (1999). Success of the modified Epley maneuver in treating benign paroxysmal positional vertigo. *Laryngoscope, 113,* 659–662.

World Health Organization (WHO). (2002). *Towards a common language for functioning, disability, and health. ICF* (pp. 1–22). Geneva, Switzerland: Author.

Yacovino, D. A., Hain, T. C., & Gualtieri, F. (2009). New therapeutic maneuver for anterior canal benign paroxysmal positional vertigo. *Journal of Neurology, 256,* 1851–1855.

Yagi, T., & Eggers, S. D. Z. (2009). Positioning and positional nystagmus testing: Background and techniques. In S. D. Z. Eggers & D. S. Zee (Eds.), *Vertigo and imbalance, clinical neurophysiology of the vestibular system* (pp. 101–110). New York, NY: Elsevier.

Zangemeister, W. H., & Bock, O. (1980). Air versus water caloric test. *Clinical Otolaryngololgy & Allied Science, 5,* 379–387.

Zapala, D. A., Olsholt, K. F., & Lundy, L. B. (2008). A comparison of water and air caloric responses and their ability to distinguish between patients with normal and impaired ears. *Ear and Hearing, 29,* 585–600.

Zigmond, A. S., & Snaith, R. P. (1983). The hospital anxiety and depression scale. *Acta Psychiatrica Scandinavica, 67,* 361–370.

Index